Mechanics of the mind

BBC Reith Lectures 1976 # Mechanics of the mind

COLIN BLAKEMORE

ROYAL SOCIETY LOCKE RESEARCH FELLOW, UNIVERSITY OF CAMBRIDGE
UNIVERSITY LECTURER IN PHYSIOLOGY
FELLOW AND DIRECTOR OF STUDIES IN MEDICINE,
DOWNING COLLEGE, CAMBRIDGE

CAMBRIDGE UNIVERSITY PRESS

CAMBRIDGE

LONDON · NEW YORK · MELBOURNE

Published by the Syndics of the Cambridge University Press
The Pitt Building, Trumpington Street, Cambridge CB2 1RP
Bentley House, 200 Euston Road, London NW1 2DB
32 East 57th Street, New York, NY 10022, USA
296 Beaconsfield Parade, Middle Park, Melbourne 3206, Australia

First published 1977
Reprinted 1977

Printed in Great Britain by
Cox & Wyman Ltd
London, Fakenham and Reading

Library of Congress Cataloguing in Publication Data

Blakemore, Colin.
Mechanics of the mind.

(BBC Reith lectures; 1976)
1. Brain – Addresses, essays, lectures.
2. Psychology, Physiological – Philosophy – Addresses,
essays, lectures. 3. Neuropsychology – Addresses,
essays, lectures. I. Title. II. Series: The Reith
lectures; 1976
QP376.B624 612.82 76–53515
ISBN 0 521 21559 5 hard covers
ISBN 0 521 29185 2 paperback

Contents

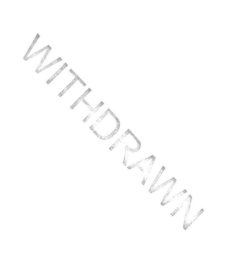

Preface

The Reith Lectures were established by the British Broadcasting Corporation in 1947; they are named for Lord Reith, founder of the BBC, in recognition of his interest in the educational value of broadcasting. I tried to forget how poorly my own experience and ability compared with those of previous lecturers and took on the task of giving the Reith Lectures in 1976 because I feel strongly that science has a duty to communicate with the society that supports it. Science done in secret (whether for reasons of national or industrial security, or because of fear of public reaction) is dangerous science. Equally, the scientist who no longer tries to communicate his ideas (either because of their incomprehensibility or because they are too specialized to be of general interest) is a poor scientist. Lord Rutherford is reputed to have told an enthusiastic but unintelligible research worker at the Cavendish Laboratory that his theories were worthless unless he could explain them to the barmaid at their local pub, 'The Bun Shop'!

Brain research is at that happy stage of science – the phase of bountiful phenomenology: the discovery of fascinating facts about the brain seems endless. Yet so much more remains to be done if we are to solve the riddle that rests within our heads and understand our minds as products of our brains. To speak in these terms is not to belittle the human mind, but to recognize it as the ultimate product of Darwinian selection, embellished by cultural evolution. The function of the brain as the instrument of human social behaviour is one of the themes of these lectures.

The text of the lectures is reproduced here in a slightly expanded form, and many illustrations have been used to supplement and build on the information in the lectures themselves.

I acknowledge here all those colleagues who helped me in the research for the lectures, or provided illustrations for this book, many of which were previously unpublished. Three people deserve special mention (if only because I know that they could each have made so much better a job of it than I have). First, Nicholas Humphrey, of the Sub-Department of Animal Behaviour, in Madingley, Cambridge, made me aware of the importance of Edward Wilson's *Sociobiology*, and steered my thoughts towards anthropology and primate ethology. Second, Gareth Matthews, of the Philosophy Department of the University of Massachusetts at Amherst, whom I had the marvellous good fortune to meet during his visit to Cambridge in 1976, taught me to begin to see the rose-coloured world through a philosopher's dark glasses. And Hendrik Van der Loos made available the excellent copy of Descartes' *Traité de l'Homme*, as well as other works in the library of the Institut d'Anatomie in Lausanne; he also read and commented on the manuscript and supplied many of the illustrations for this book.

In addition, Laurence Garey and Mark Haggard each read and criticized parts of the manuscript; David Paterson, the Producer of the lectures, gave me a great deal of help; Sarah Waters researched the illustrations with superb skill and amazing speed; and Andrée Blakemore was always the first and therefore the most influential critic, and also helped to translate the *Ballade* by François Villon.

Cambridge, 1977   C. B.

TO HENRY M.

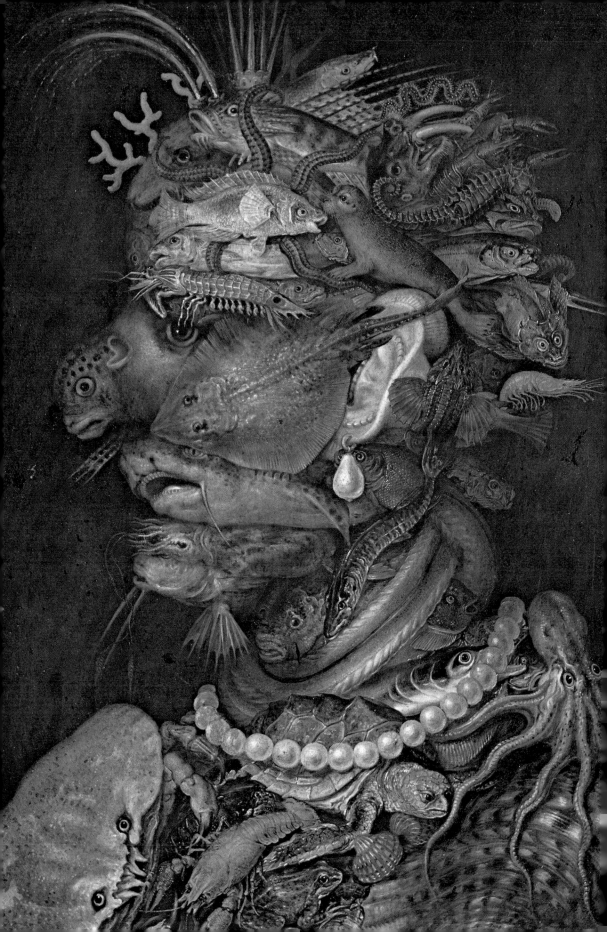

1 The divinest part of us

Copying the round shape of the universe, they confined the two divine revolutions in a spherical body – the head, as we now call it – which is the divinest part of us and lord over all the rest.

Plato, *Timaeus*

1848 was a year of revolution in Europe; Karl Marx and Friedrich Engels published the *Communist Manifesto*, and political demonstrations tore apart the great cities of Paris, Vienna, Naples and Berlin. That same year, in New England, a bizarre accident touched off a minor revolution of a different sort – not a radical change in man's attitude to man, but a turning point in his understanding of that part of man which fosters social conscience – his mind.

The accident occurred at about half past four in the afternoon of 13 September 1848 near the small town of Cavendish, Vermont. A gang of men, under the direction of their energetic and likeable foreman, 25-year-old Phineas P. Gage, was working on the new line of the Rutland and Burlington Railroad. They were about to blast a rock that blocked their way and Phineas himself took charge of the delicate business of pouring gunpowder into a deep narrow hole drilled in the stone. The powder in place, he rammed in a long iron rod to tamp down the charge before covering it with sand. But the tamping iron rubbed against the side of the shaft and a spark ignited the powder. The massive rod, three and a half feet long, an inch and a quarter in diameter, weigh-

'Water' by Giuseppe Arcimboldo (1527–1593).

I

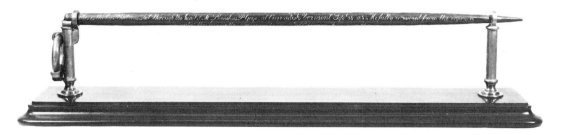

The tamping iron of Phineas Gage is now kept at Harvard University. On it is engraved: 'This is the bar that was shot through the head of Mr Phinelius P. Gage at Cavendish, Vermont, Sept. 14, 1848. He fully recovered from the injure & deposited this bar in the Museum of the Medical College, Harvard University.'

ing thirteen pounds, shot from the hole under the force of the explosion. This terrible missile struck Phineas Gage just beneath his left eye and, in a fraction of time, tore through his skull, departed from a hole in the top of his head, and finally landed some fifty yards away.

Believe it or not, that was not the end of Phineas P. Gage – at least not of the body that bore his name. He was thrown to the ground, and his hands and feet twitched convulsively; but within a few minutes he was conscious again, and able to speak. The other workmen carried him gently to an ox-cart nearby and he rode for three quarters of a mile, sitting upright, to a hotel in the town. With little assistance he stepped from the cart, climbed a long flight of stairs to a room where his awful injuries were dressed and he awaited the arrival of the local physicians. The two doctors could hardly believe the incredible tale until, like Doubting Thomas, they examined his wounds with their own hands.

At ten o'clock that same evening, though the bleeding was still terrible, Phineas was rational enough to say that he did not need to see his friends because he should be back to work within a couple of days. There could be no doubt that a large metal rod had passed completely through the part of his brain that filled his forehead, yet his senses and speech were normal and his memory apparently unimpaired.

The next few days were difficult. The wound became infected and Phineas was anaemic and delirious. But with liberal doses of calomel, rhubarb and castor oil he slowly improved and after three weeks he called for his trousers and was eager to escape from his bed. By the middle of November he was wandering about the town, planning his new future. And here is the point of this curious tale. Phineas Gage had a *new* future for he was a different man. The efficient and capable foreman no longer existed; the friendly, considerate Phineas Gage was dead, and in his place rose a child-like Phoenix with the strength of an ox and an evil temper to match it.

Years later, John Harlow, one of the two doctors who had originally attended him, wrote:

'His physical health is good, and I am inclined to say that he has recovered . . . The equilibrium or balance, so to speak, between his intellectual faculties and animal propensities, seems to have been destroyed. He is fitful, irreverent, indulging at times in the grossest profanity (which was not previously his custom), manifesting but little deference for his fellows, impatient of restraint or advice when it conflicts with his desires, at times pertinaciously obstinate, yet capricious and vacillating, devis-

Phineas Gage's skull bears the marks of his unique injury. The displaced flap of bone grew to cover partly the hole above his frontal lobes. Beside the skull is a life mask of Mr Gage.

ing many plans of future operation, which are no sooner arranged than they are abandoned . . . In this regard his mind was radically changed, so decidedly that his friends and acquaintances said that he was "no longer Gage".'

The new Phineas Gage was rejected by his previous employers and he drifted around the United States and South America exhibiting himself, and the tamping iron that had twisted his mind, as a fairground attraction. He died in San Francisco, but his skull and iron rod are still on display to the public, in the museum of Harvard Medical School.

News of the metamorphosis of Phineas Gage reached the ears of the medical world in the 1860s; and it could not have come at a more crucial time. It seemed the final

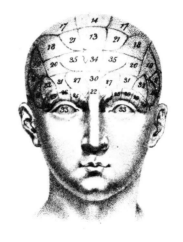

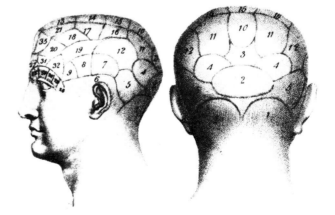

The early system of phrenological classification of bumps on the skull was quite modest. Gall himself named twenty-seven 'organs' and his enthusiastic colleague, Johann Caspar Spurzheim (1776–1832), also a competent dissector, added eight more localized faculties. These drawings are from a book published by Spurzheim in 1825.

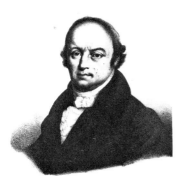

piece to the jigsaw puzzle of the mind. The idea that different mental functions are localized in various parts of the tissue of the brain was becoming a dominant one. The rapid historical movement towards this opinion was started by a long-discredited Viennese physician, Franz Joseph Gall. As a boy, Gall had noticed that a number of acquaintances with particularly good memories also had large, protruding eyes. 'I was forced to the idea', he wrote in 1812, 'that eyes so formed are the mark of an excellent memory . . . Why should not the other faculties also have their visible external characteristics?' 'From this time all the individuals who were distinguished by any quality or faculty became the object of my special attention, and of systematic study as to the form of the head.'

Gall travelled to foundling homes, prisons and lunatic

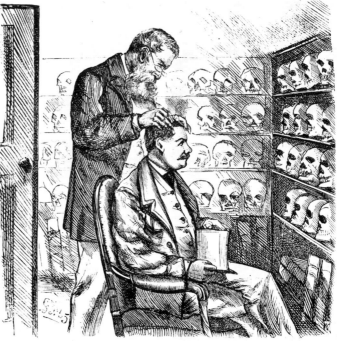

A HINT TO PHRENOLOGISTS; or, "September 20, 1878."

OPERATOR IN STOCKS (*who desires a chart of his head, interrogatively*). "I say, Professor, it occurs to me, from the number of skulls I see, that you will have rather a lively time in this Establishment on Resurrection-Day?"

PROFESSOR (*who can find no traces of the bump of veneration*). "No; we shouldn't anticipate any trouble, except, perhaps, from those Wall Street Skulls on the second shelf: they might appropriate other people's bones, and create a temporary panic."

Almost from its inception phrenology was the subject of ridicule by many scientists (as was the theory of natural selection). By the middle of the eighteenth century it was a popular theme in jokes and cartoons.

5

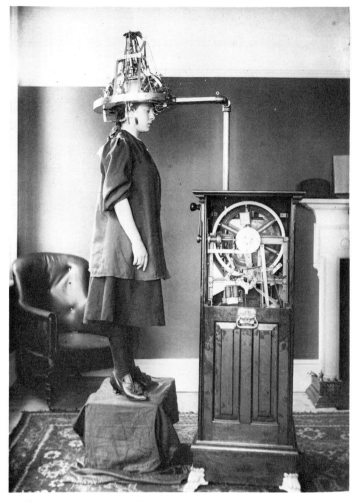

Phrenology died a slow death. The Lavery Electric Phrenometer of 1907 was intended to lend twentieth-century accuracy to the measurement of bumps. As late as 1938 there was an Ohio State Phrenological Society, which published its own journal, and the British Phrenological Society was not disbanded until 1967.

asylums in his search for people with extraordinary heads, and built up a huge anecdotal catalogue of the relationship between particular mental characteristics and bumps on the skull, including an especially amorous ladyfriend with exceptional protuberances behind her ears. Armed with this motley index of skull bumps, Gall conceived the theory of phrenology. He argued that all the faculties of the mind, even moral and intellectual, are inherited in each person, a view received quite sympathetically by early Victorian society. Moreover, each characteristic must be controlled by a separate, innately localized 'organ', within the great cerebral hemispheres

6

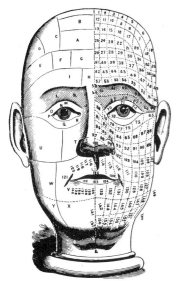

J. W. Redfield, MD, of New York, published this extraordinary diagram in 1894. It combines physiognomy, the classification of facial characteristics, with a kind of 'micro-phrenology'. Amongst the 160 numbered faculties is No. 149: 'Republicanism'.

of the brain, directly under the skull. This pseudo-science was an ungainly child, fruit of the union between inchoate anatomy and the Romantic movement, with its fascination for the analysis of character.

An analogy can be drawn between the scientific methods of the phrenologists and Charles Darwin's purely descriptive evidence for his theory of natural selection. But unlike the hypothesis of evolution, phrenology was a band-wagon riding on a bumpy road to scientific disgrace; it was entertained seriously only until the middle of the last century. But it did shift the paradigm of science, in the terminology of Thomas Kuhn, and prepared the way for the studies of great neurologists in London and Paris. They observed the symptoms of human patients who had suffered circumscribed damage to parts of the cerebral hemispheres, and suggested that the control of movement, the sensations and even the power of speech *were* strictly localized in the brain.

Phineas Gage cemented this new phrenology. Even the imponderable elements of the mind, responsibility, personality and compassion must have their machinery in the brain – in the frontal lobes that had been torn apart by the iron rod.

One of the many valuable outcomes of the phrenological movement was an increased interest, amongst anatomists, in the cerebral cortex. Before the last century the cortex itself (now believed to be the seat of most of the 'higher' functions of the brain) was rarely represented with accuracy in anatomical illustrations. This diagram of 1830, by L. Rolando, shows the right cerebral hemispheres of the human brain. The convoluted surface of the cerebral cortex is accurately drawn, but the numbers refer to the phrenological 'organs'.

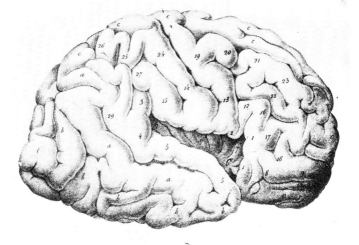

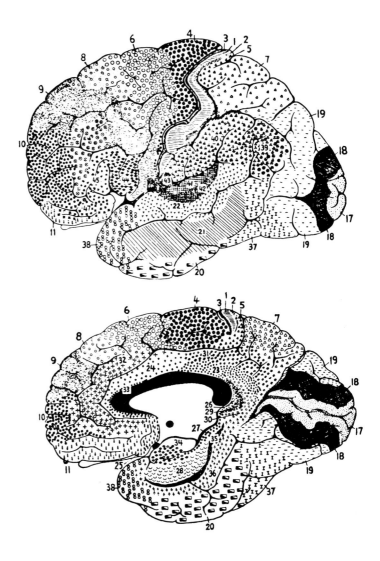

The advent of improved methods of sectioning and staining very thin slices of the brain, at the end of the last century, led to the classification of cortical areas on the basis of differences (sometimes very subtle) in their microscopic appearance. Korbinian Brodmann (1868–1918) was perhaps the best-known practitioner of 'cytoarchitectonics'. This is his 1909 map of the human cortex: above is a side-view of the left hemisphere, and below a view of the right hemisphere from the inside, after the brain has been split in half down the midline. Brodmann's numbers are still widely used, even though some would criticize this approach as not much more than neo-phrenology!

Of course, the relationship between injuries to the head and insult to the mind was hardly a new discovery in the nineteenth century. Even the Hippocratic School of physicians, who, four hundred years before Christ, first challenged the ancient supernatural concepts of illness, knew that the Sacred Disease of epilepsy, and madness itself, were disturbances of the brain. They went so far as to say:

'Not only our pleasure, our joy and our laughter but also our sorrow, pain, grief and tears arise from the brain, and the brain alone. With it we think and understand, see and hear, and we discriminate between the ugly and the beautiful, between what is pleasant and what is unpleasant and between good and evil.'

While such a materialistic statement would be a perfectly acceptable preface to a modern textbook on the brain, it was not generally accepted in ancient times. The disagreement was not, however, about the materialistic assumptions that sustained such speculation; perhaps the brain of man is best fitted for dealing with material things, even when considering his own mental functions. The debate that raged, since at least the time that men first wrote down those things that troubled them, was not about *whether* the mind had a physical counterpart in the body, but *where* its embodiment might be.

It seems almost inconceivable today that anyone could ever doubt that man's mind is in his brain. For me, the 'me-ness' of me is undoubtedly situated about two inches behind my eyes, in the very middle of my head. But I am sure that I feel this with such confidence because I accept the currently fashionable scientific evidence that it is so.

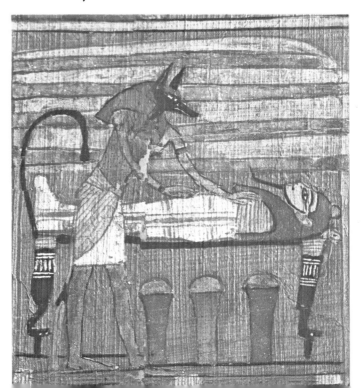

Anubis, the Heavenly Embalmer, prepares a mummified corpse. Detail from a Book of the Dead from File, Egypt, c. 1250 B.C.

To the ancient Egyptians it was definitely somewhere else, for though they entombed their dead leaders with all the tangible trappings of life and tried to preserve in perfect condition their bodily remains for the journey to Osiris, they dealt summarily with the brain by retracting it through the nose with a spoon. The Ba spirit of an Egyptian mummy was not in his head, but in his bowels and his heart.

At one time or another almost every major organ in the body has been credited with this ultimate organic privilege – the guardianship of the soul and of the sentiments that make us men. The liver, blood-coloured and apparently the source of all the veins, played this special role for the Sumerians (the first people to write down their thoughts), for the Assyrians and for the ancient people of Israel. 'My liver shall sing praise to Thee, and not be silent', the Psalmist may literally have written.

It is hardly surprising that the arrangement of blood vessels should have guided man in his search for his soul. After all, what is a soul? It is a mover, an animator (that word itself is derived from 'anima', the Latin for 'soul'). And what could be more necessary for the sustenance of movement than the free flow of warming blood through the body. When blood was lost, then so was life. By this argument, the origin of blood must be the source of life itself, and from this view sprang one of the most enduring theories of biology – that the seat of the soul is the heart. Aristotle himself, the greatest biologist in the ancient world, supported this idea, and it is still with us; not in science perhaps, but certainly in poetry and in popular song, where the heart, not the brain, yearns, aches and finally breaks.

Aristotle's specific theory relegated the brain to the task of merely cooling blood from the heart, which was itself the organ of thought and sensation. Aristotle's great gift to science was the method of observation. In this particular case his own conclusions were wrong, but

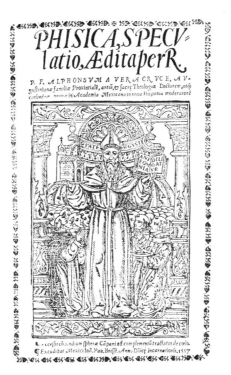

PHISICA,SPECV
latio,ÆditaperR.

Aristotle (384–322 B.C.). From the frontispiece of Phisica Speculatio *by Alonso de la Veracruz (1504–1584), published in Mexico in 1557; the first scientific book published in America.*

by dissecting and describing what he saw, he questioned the value of speculation based on pure reason and hence invented the scientific method.

Like every good student, Aristotle had grown wise enough to know when his teacher was wrong. He had been a student of Plato, who himself studied with Socrates and founded the great Academy in Athens in about 387 B.C. Plato virtually rejected experiment and even observation. He argued that, since our senses so obviously deceive us, they are not to be trusted; true knowledge comes only from pure thought, unadulterated by evidence. Mystical contemplation and the methods of mathematics can discover the truth of everything. So Plato did not dissect, and only acquired information about the body second-hand from the Greek scholars of medicine living in southern Italy. Yet it was Plato, not Aristotle, who championed the brain as the seat of the soul. If it was not genuine scientific evidence that led Plato to this choice, then what did? The answer can be found in the social, political and cultural context in which he lived.

Plato was a wealthy aristocrat who believed that leisure was essential to wisdom, which was therefore automatically denied to the working poor. In Plato's utopian world, described in his *Republic*, society would be utterly hierarchical, with absolute power by cultural inheritance in the hands of a minority of philosophers, the Guardians. And just as the senses (the guardians of the body) could lie, so could the government of Plato's Republic. His concept of the universe, and of man's mind within it, was no less structured and hierarchical than his idealized intellectual oligarchy. Without experiment and without empirical knowledge, Plato postulated that the spiritual mind of man, the rational soul, is in his head. He believed that mathematics is the essential mode of thought, and it was mathematics that led him to succeed where Aristotle had failed in deciding the location of the mind. The perfect geometrical shape, he argued, is a sphere: the spherical earth rests within the globes of the heavens, and at the centre of the entire living Cosmos of Plato stands man (the philosopher, of course). Where else could it be, the rational soul, 'the divinest part of us', as Plato called it, but in the spherical head, the summit of the human body?

Plato had another reason for choosing the head, a reason of much greater interest to the scientist. He was trying to solve the central conundrum in biology – the mystery of inheritance. To justify Plato's political concept of eugenically controlled status in society, he proposed that a philosopher-king is likely to pass to his children the elements of his rational mind, as well as the appearance of his body. Plato saw a similarity between the substance of the brain itself and male semen.

Greek society at the time had little part for woman to play: she was but a flowerpot for the seed of man, which (by Plato's account) was derived from his brain. Although Plato proposed equality for women in the intellectual competition of his idealized Republic, he was usually less generous to her, for instance when discussing the transmigration of souls in his dialogue *The Timaeus*. If a man lived well, and overcame his animal emotions, he would, after death, be reborn in a star. If not he would suffer the ignominy of re-creation as a woman. If *she* lived badly, the wretched soul would find itself in an animal.

Persistence of the soul beyond mere physical death is an almost universal tenet of religions and philosophies. It is not, I believe, an expression of man's selfishness alone; it is the inevitable cultural formulation of the most basic and most essential requirement of any living thing – the desire to survive. In Darwin's theory it was amply fulfilled by successful and abundant self-reproduction. To the egocentric Platonists, re-incarnation was needed too.

The free movement of souls within Plato's anthropocentric universe was possible because the Cosmos itself was alive. Pre-Newtonian mechanics demanded that anything that moves must have a mover; the heavens themselves are in motion and therefore must be moved by a cosmic soul. Animals and plants must also have souls, though lesser souls than the rational soul of man, and so too must the very substance of the earth. The current interest in the defence of the environment and the attempt to establish legal rights for mountain, wilderness and recreation areas is, in a sense, a return to a Platonic view of the living Cosmos.

Transmigration of the soul is not, however, an idea original to Plato, nor is his the most extreme example of the hypothesis. Pythagoras, who probably founded geometry with his theorem about the dimensions of right-angled triangles, thought that in a previous existence he had been a bush! The religious philosophy of the Pythagorean brotherhood seems laughable today; two of their strict rules were that one should pick up nothing that had been dropped, and that no one should ever eat beans! However, as Bertrand Russell wrote, 'Beginnings are apt to be crude, but their originality should not be overlooked on this account.' The rules of the Pythagorean order were based on their fascination with the mysticism of numbers and geometry. Though naive, this was the beginning of the fusion of science and everyday life.

There is even more reason to emphasize the importance of ancient Greek views about the mechanism of mentality, particularly those of Plato and Aristotle. For their opinions and their authority, sanctified and dogmatized by the early Christian fathers, became the unquestionable truth that shackled the mind of man in the Middle Ages and slowed the advance of civilization to a hesitant crawl. By its monopoly of what little education there was, the Church cultivated and perpetuated an extraordinary model of the mind that grew in complexity and richness, not by further observation or even by genuine debate, but by the barren science of endlessly interpreting classical ideas. An incongruous marriage was arranged between the theories of Plato and Aristotle and biblical dogma. It reconciled heart-centred and brain-centred views of the mind by incorporating both organs in a great cognitive waterworks. Nutrients, absorbed from the intestines, passed to the liver where a fluid called *natural spirit* was formed; this flowed to the heart where it became *vital spirit* which pulsed towards a marvellous network of blood vessels, the *rete mirabile*, at the base of the brain. Here it mixed with air inspired through the nose into the porous base of the skull. The final product was a perfect distillation, called *animal spirit* (again from the Latin, 'anima'), which was stored in the system of fluid-filled cavities, the ventricles, running through the entire brain. This spirit, formed from the mixture of liquid and air, was the

14

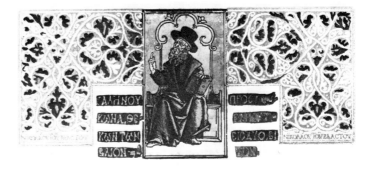

essence of life and the source of all intellect. Could W. B. Yeats have had this in mind when he said of a poem, 'I made it out of a mouthful of air'?

The arrangement of the brain ventricles was known from the observations of the great Greek anatomist Galen of Bergama in the second century A.D., as interpreted by an eleventh-century Persian writer, Ibn Sina

This drawing appeared in 1496, in Epitomate *by Gerardus de Harderwyck. The lower figure has his head symbolically divided into the three 'cellulae' of the ventricular doctrine. Into the first cell, containing the 'sensus communis', come signals from the ears, eyes, nose, tongue and skin. As a gesture to the Aristotelian theory, the heart is also given importance; it too is connected with the ears and the brain. The upper pair of heads illustrate alternative four-cell and five-cell schemes.*

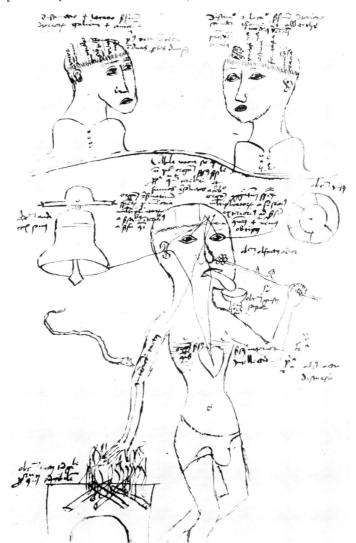

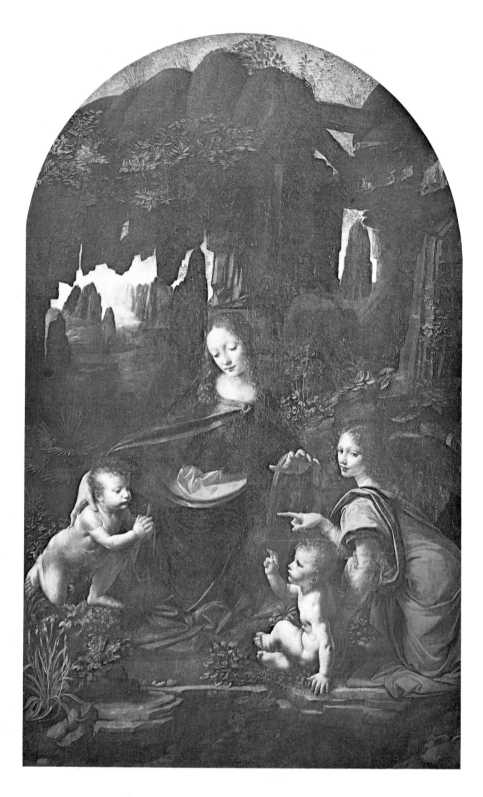

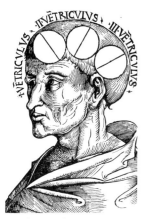

The ventricular system was represented in a highly symbolic form in many medieval drawings. This one is from the 1506 edition of the Philosophia pauperum of Albertus Magnus (1206–1280).

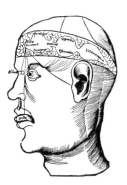

This cell diagram, published in 1503 by Gregor Reisch, was one of the most popular and it was copied by many subsequent authors. The first cell is inscribed 'Sensus communis', 'imaginativa' and 'fantasia', the second 'cogitatia' and 'estimatia', and the third 'memorativa'.

◄

Perhaps because of his brilliance as an artist, Leonardo's scientific findings, some of them original and revolutionary, had little influence on the history of science. 'La Vergine delle rocce' by Leonardo da Vinci.

or Avicenna. There are four ventricles but the first two form a symmetrical pair within the large cerebral hemispheres at the front of the brain. They communicate with the middle ventricle in the forebrain, which connects through a narrow canal with the last ventricle in the stem of the brain. This system of three connected compartments, the front pair, the middle and the last, allowed the medievalists to give tangible form to one of Plato's important ideas, that the action of the mind proceeds through a series of operations, from sensation to memory. The first pair of ventricles was said to be the site of the *sensus communis*, the mechanism of sensory analysis, which was connected with the nerve of the sense organs. Here images were created and passed on to the middle ventricle, which was the seat of reason (*ratio*), thought (*cognatio*) or judgement (*aestimatio*). The final step was memory itself (*memoria*), in the last ventricle.

This remarkable scheme persisted in written accounts and illustrations until the seventeenth century, but it began to be questioned, as did so many areas of scientific authority, in the Renaissance. Two men in particular broke the barriers of superstition, slipping the progress of knowledge into higher gear. They were that symbol of the Renaissance, Leonardo da Vinci, and the seventeenth-century founder of modern philosophy, René Descartes.

Leonardo is not distinguished principally as a scientist, nor as a mathematician, an engineer, an architect, or even an artist. His most remarkable achievement, and the thing that makes him more than anyone a Renaissance man, is the fact that he was *all* of these. He had what is essential for progress in art no less than in science – disbelief. He did not believe that things could not be done, nor that they *should* not be done, because they had not been done before. 'I wish to work miracles,' he said. 'I may have fewer possessions than other men who are

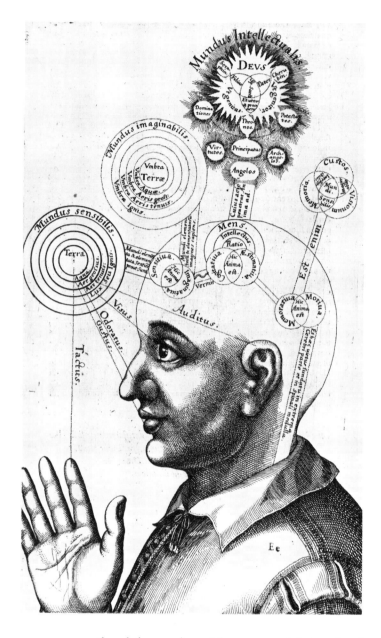

The intricate orbits of the mind in this drawing by the Paracelsian mystic, Robert Fludd (1574–1637), are based on the classic three-cell model. From Utriusque Cosmi, 1619–1621.

more tranquil and those who wish to grow rich in a day.' But his temerity and disregard for dogma brought him into conflict with the Church, just as it did Galileo. 'Whoever in discussion,' wrote Leonardo, 'adduces authority uses not his intellect but rather memory.' 'Science comes by observation, not by authority.'

In no field of endeavour was Leonardo's dispute with the Church more bitter than in his anatomical studies. To dissect the human body was not only to question the absolute authority of the descriptions of Galen and Avicenna, but also to abuse the sanctity of the human corpse. But Leonardo did dissect, both to learn how to make better drawings and to understand the nature of the body as a perfect machine. News of his experiments caused the Pope to withdraw his favour and Leonardo was compelled to leave Rome in 1515.

Now, in about 1490, Leonardo had drawn anatomical illustrations of the human head and brain that incorporated the classical ventricular scheme, with the nerves from the eyes connecting to the *sensus communis* in the first chamber. But curiosity prevailed and some time between 1504 and 1507 he performed a detailed dissection of the brain of an ox. But how can one dissect a system of cavities? The ventricles are only defined by the absence of brain tissue. Leonardo overcame this problem

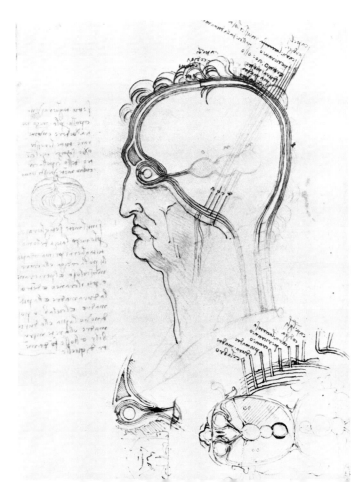

Leonardo drew these beautiful but inaccurate pictures of the ventricles in 1490. In the lower horizontal section through the head he shows the optic nerves, from the eyes, converging on to the first ventricle.

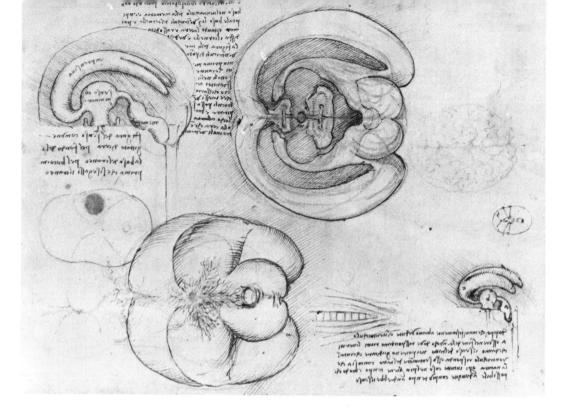

with typical originality: he injected the ventricles of the brain with molten wax, waited for it to set and dissected the tissue away from what remained – the first cast of the ventricles. No doubt Leonardo's experience with casting statues in bronze had prompted this brilliant strategy. (The technique of filling the human ventricles with air is used today in the preparation of X-ray pictures of the brain, showing the shapes of the ventricles in disease.)

What Leonardo saw forced him to reorchestrate the classical description of serial processing in the brain

By about 1506, Leonardo had made a wax cast of the ventricles. He wrote 'senso commune' not on the banana-shaped first pair of ventricles, but on the middle one.

Computerized X-ray axial tomography is the latest method of exploring the shape and distortion of the human brain and its ventricles. A British invention, the EMI scanner, uses a fine X-ray beam and a ring of sensitive detectors, which are rotated around the head. A computer builds up a cross-sectional picture of the head, with remarkable resolution. The colours indicate different densities of tissue. This patient, a 79-year-old woman, had been admitted to hospital in a drowsy state after two falls. The red area on the right is a blood clot lying on the brain.

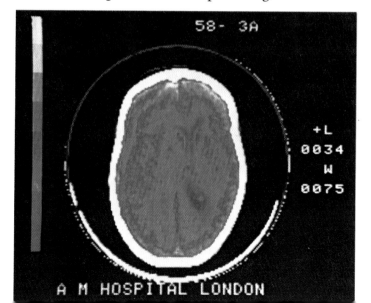

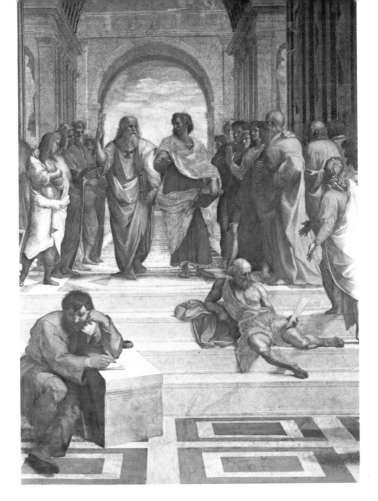

'The School of Athens' by Raphael.

which had originated with Plato. He found that many of the nerves from the sense organs did not arrive near the anterior pair of ventricles, but in the tissue, now called the *thalamus*, around the middle ventricle. Even Leonardo did not have the courage to leap from the conceptual cliff. The illustration that he drew was accurate in form but the names that he used to label the parts were classical ones. He insisted, however, on moving the *sensus communis* to the middle ventricle, which in the classical scheme had been occupied by the power of judgement. It is possible that we owe to Leonardo our current usage of the phrase *common sense* to mean reason and judgement!

Though his influence on scientific thought was slight, Leonardo had, symbolically, broken Plato's death grip

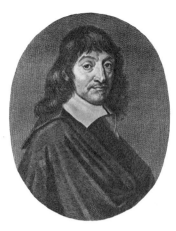

René Descartes (1596–1650).

on the science of the mind. In about 1510, Raphael, a contemporary of Leonardo, painted his magnificent mural devoted to Philosophy in the Stanza della Segnatura, in the Vatican. It shows Plato's Academy in Athens, and in the centre, by the figure of Aristotle, stands Plato himself, with a copy of *The Timaeus* in his hands. Many historians of art believe that Raphael used, as his model for Plato, Leonardo da Vinci himself; certainly the resemblance to late self-portraits by Leonardo is striking. What irony that he should have chosen Leonardo to represent the very man whose authority Leonardo so much disliked.

René Descartes' special contribution was not empirical but conceptual. Like Plato, he doubted the reliability of his senses and, indeed, in 1637 he proposed that the only admissible approach to the establishment of knowledge was to disregard all beliefs about which he had the slightest doubt. The first thing he found that he could *not* doubt was his own existence as a purely thinking thing: '*Cogito ergo sum*'.

Descartes made a radical distinction between a mind (something known to itself with immediate certainty) and a body (something whose very existence must be inferred from experience). By its nature the human body, even the entire nervous system, was a mere machine. In this respect there was nothing to distinguish between man and beast.

In the *Traité de l'Homme*, Descartes wrote, with a material frankness that might have shocked even behavioural psychologists earlier this century:

'I wish you to consider, finally, that all the functions which I attribute to this machine, such as digestion . . . nutrition . . . respiration, waking and sleeping; the reception of light, sounds, odours . . ., the impression of ideas in the organ of the common sense and imagination; the retention of these ideas in the memory; the

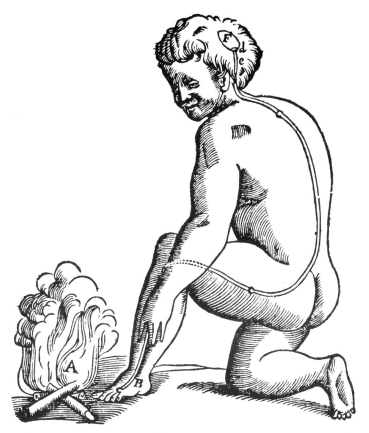

Not least of Descartes' achievements was his introduction of the concept of the automatic 'reflex' as an extension of the Aristotelian and Medieval ideas of a hydraulic system of spirit. In this example, the fire (A) is said to 'have force enough to displace the area of skin, . . . thus pulling the tiny thread CC, which you see to be attached there . . . just as, pulling on one end of a cord, one simultaneously rings a bell which hangs at the opposite end'. The pull on the cord (the sensory nerves from the skin) opens a pore (d) in the ventricle (F) of the brain, allowing animal spirit to flow out of the ventricle through what Descartes saw as hollow tubes in the centres of the nerves connecting to the muscles of the leg. The spirit inflates the muscles, causing the foot (B) to withdraw. Other motor nerves are also operated, making the eyes and head turn towards the foot, and the hands and the whole body move to protect the injured part.

inferior movements of the appetites and passions; and finally the movements of all the external members . . .; I desire, I say, that you consider that these functions occur naturally in this machine solely by the disposition of its organs, not less than the movements of a clock.'

Descartes had split the body and the mind, but certainly did not abandon the latter. He was a devout Catholic and had even decided against publishing his theory of an infinite universe when he heard of the first condemnation of Galileo in 1616. No; for Descartes the rational soul or mind was the only thing that separated man from the animals. He even found an anatomical point of contact between the soul and the body – the pea-sized pineal gland, an enigmatic pimple on the back of the brain whose true function is still uncertain.

23

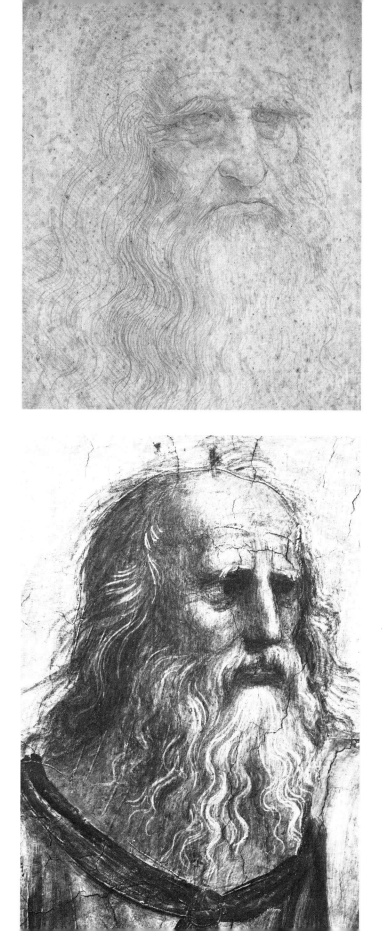

A late self-portrait of Leonardo, from the Biblioteca Reale, Turin.

Plato; detail from 'The School of Athens'.

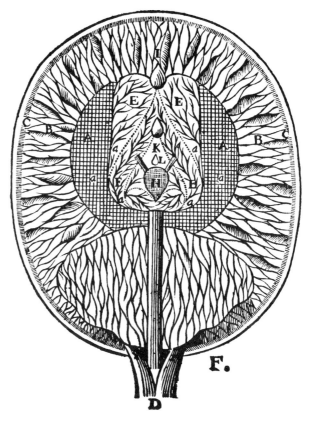

Descartes was not concerned to represent structure accurately in this diagram of the brain (which is reminiscent of the geometric abstraction of the anatomical illustrations of the Arabs, who were forbidden to represent the human form). He was more interested in illustrating models of the function of the brain. He thought of the pineal gland (H), the tear-shaped organ in the middle of the head, as the major source of animal spirit, derived from the arteries. This spirit is secreted into the ventricle (E–E) and makes its way out through the meshwork of tiny pores (a) in the walls of the ventricle (A). The threads (B), running from the walls of the ventricle down into the spinal cord (D), can be bent into new shapes by the force of the spirit flowing out through the pores between them, down towards the muscles. Inclination of the pineal gland in different directions (at the whim of the soul) can cause 'voluntary' changes in the distribution of spirit to the muscles.

Descartes' achievement was to make explicit the principle of *dualism*, that the bodily functions of the brain are entirely distinct from the mystical domain of the soul. Dualism has served its purpose, though it still haunts the terminology of brain research and feeds the common belief that there is some magic in the mind. But in its time, dualism was a liberating dictum; it freed men, even devout men, to speculate about the working substance of the brain, without fear of treading in the footprints of God. It made possible the co-existence of sincere belief in a rational soul and a materialistic attitude towards the mundane part of the mind.

Nothing illustrates better the constraint that man's view of his own cultural position in society places on the way that he analyses Nature through science. The historical evolution of the concept of the mind mirrors

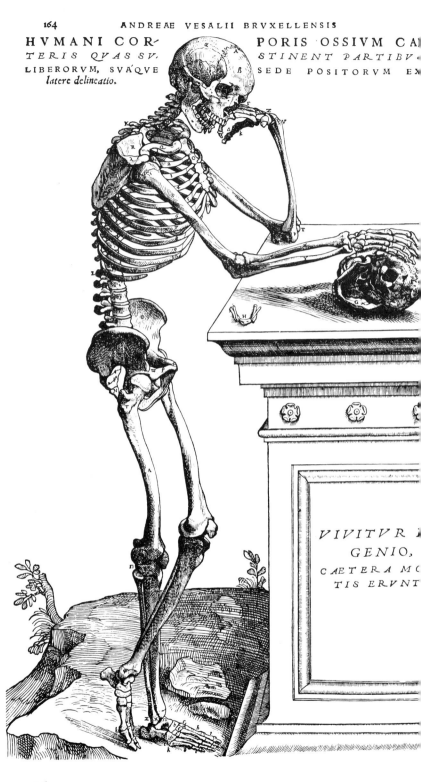

HVMANI COR-   PORIS OSSIVM CA
TERIS QVAS SV.   *STINENT PARTIBV*
LIBERORVM, SVA'QVE   SEDE POSITORVM EX
latere delineatio.

*VIVITVR
GENIO,
CAETERA MO
TIS ERVNT*

*A skeleton contemplates a skull.
From De Fabrica (1543) by
Andreas Vesalius, perhaps the
greatest anatomist of all time.*

26

man's social development, from Plato's genetically controlled meritocracy of the mind, to Gall's picture of innate organs of intelligence and character shining through the honesty of the shape of a man's head. The force is still with us. Current debates about the inheritance of intelligence, about the use of techniques of behavioural modification and about the genetic basis of social behaviour show that *our* models of the mind are still a part of the political and social theory by which we live.

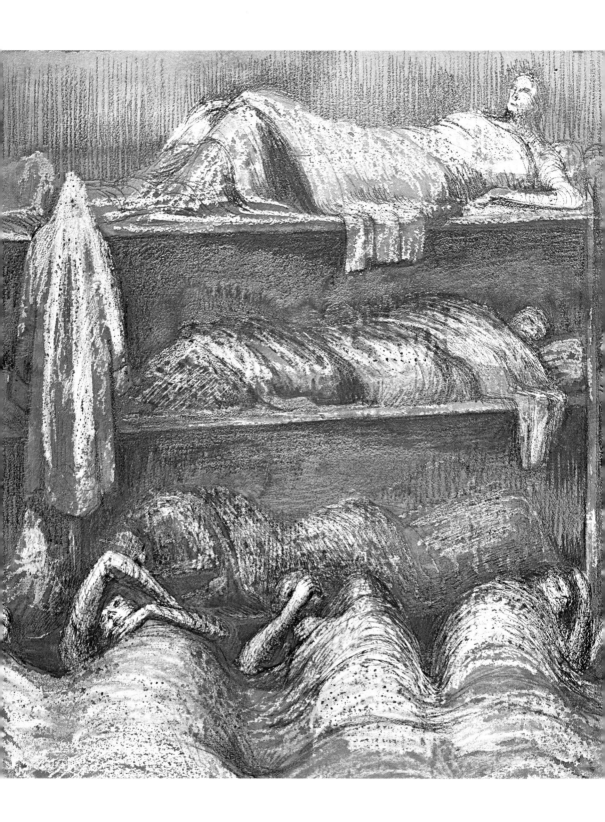

2 Chuang Tzu and the butterfly

O the mind, mind has mountains; cliffs of fall
Frightful, sheer, no-man-fathomed. Hold them cheap
May who ne'er hung there. Nor does long our small
Durance deal with that steep or deep. Here! creep,
Wretch, under a comfort serves in a whirlwind: all
Life death does end and each day dies with sleep.

Gerard Manley Hopkins (1844–1889)

Nathaniel Kleitman, a Russian emigré who settled in the United States in 1915, and Bruce Richardson, an American colleague, spent thirty-two days alone in the depths of Mammoth Cave, Kentucky, in 1938. They were completely isolated from information about the state of the outside world, suspended in an unchanging microcosm: constant temperature, constant humidity. Only the artificial lights in their underground home preserved the rhythmic cycles of the day. But the day by which Kleitman and Richardson lived was not the day of this earth. They forced themselves to join the routine of an unknown planet, one with a twenty-eight hour day, nineteen hours for waking and nine for sleep. Could their bodies tolerate this sudden space-flight to a world of different time? Kleitman, a pioneer of the scientific study of sleep at the University of Chicago, had already developed methods of measuring continually the normal fluctuations of body temperature (hotter in the early afternoon, cooler in the early morning), and of recording the tossing and turning of restless sleep. He used the same techniques in Mammoth Cave to see

◀
'Shelter Scene, Sleepers', 1975, by
Henry Moore.

29

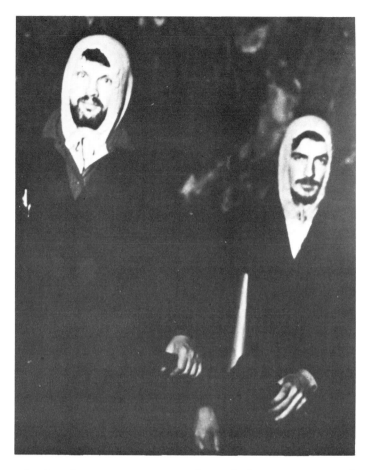

Nathaniel Kleitman and Bruce Richardson leaving Mammoth Cave in 1938.

whether his temperature cycle and sleep pattern, and those of Richardson, his companion, would stick to earth-time or switch to the clock of Planet X. To be brief, Kleitman stuck and Richardson switched! Kleitman was unable to adjust to the twenty-eight-hour day: his body temperature stubbornly followed the rhythm of the world outside the cave and his sleep was inadequate and fitful, especially when, every six days, 'midnight' in the cave coincided with noon in the real Kentucky. Richardson, on the other hand, adapted well in his temperature cycle and his sleep pattern.

Similar experiments in underground bunkers in Germany and in the continuous daylight of summer in the Arctic Circle have proved that man has a clock in his brain – set to the time cycle of his natural home. On their flights to the moon the American astronauts took with them not only quotations from the 'Bible and a collapsible American flag, but also this mental chronometer, which reminded them of Houston wherever they went. They slept, shaved and ate on their own earth-time. Like a real clock, the brain's clock can readily be shifted back or forth, but with some discomfort to its owner, as every jet traveller knows. Again, like a real clock, there is less scope for speeding it up or slowing it down; Bruce Richardson was one of the rare individuals who can tolerate a regular twenty-eight-hour day; most of us can only manage between twenty-two and twenty-six.

Man is certainly not unique in having internal knowledge of the periodicity of time; even the simplest multicellular sea animals have their cycles of activity locked to the rotation of the earth on its axis. And the humble rat stirs from its daytime sleep at precisely the same time each evening; the rules of the solar system may be written in its genetic code. A rat kept in a room that is constantly dark or continuously illuminated will still obey a cycle of activity, but usually with a natural periodicity a little longer than twenty-four hours. It will

These graphs, based on measurements made in Mammoth Cave, show how Bruce Richardson adjusted well in his body temperature cycle but Nathaniel Kleitman did not. Their body temperatures went up and down rhythmically and Richardson's became locked to the artificial 28-hour day; it had only six peaks during the six artificial days in this diagram. On the other hand, Kleitman's graph had seven peaks, which always coincided with early afternoon outside the cave, as shown by the calendar on the bottom line. The shaded areas indicate the nine-hour periods spent in bed. Kleitman slept particularly badly during the third sleep period, because it coincided with the peak in his body temperature.

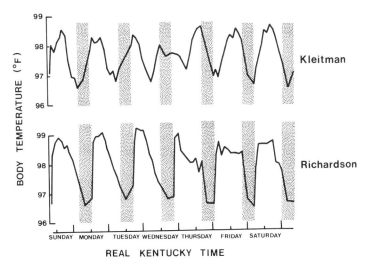

31

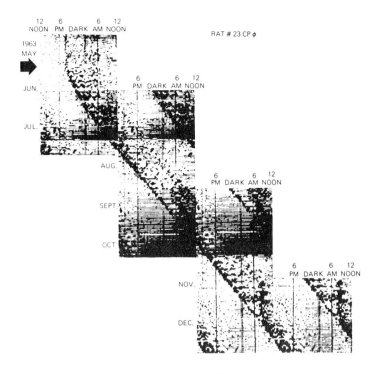

The daily cycle of activity of a rat is recorded over an eight month period. Each horizontal line represents a 24-hour day running from noon one day to noon the next day; the line thickens whenever the rat moves about. At first, the period of most activity occurs regularly during the night, between about 8 p.m. and 6 a.m. Early in May, at the point shown by the large arrow, the rat was suddenly deprived of all information about the natural 24-hour light–dark cycle. Despite this it continued its cyclical period of activity but with a rhythm of just a few minutes longer than 24 hours; so the repetitive pattern of darkening on the record is not exactly locked to the 24-hour day, and drifts, like a real clock running slightly slowly. The natural cycle is, however, extremely regular: the slope of the dark band is constant for more than seven months. Results of Curt Richter (1967).

not deviate from this inherent rhythm by more than a few minutes over several months; the time-keeper in a rat's brain is more accurate than most mechanical clocks.

In laboratories all over the world, the study of human sleep remains the most direct experimental approach to the question of consciousness. This nightly appointment with death is the most profound loss of consciousness that most of us are likely to experience throughout our lives. We shall spend more than twenty years of our lifetime asleep, unconscious, almost oblivious to the demands, the joys, the dangers of the world around us.

The problem of human consciousness has stirred up fierce debate between the reductionists, who would banish the Cartesian soul from the machinery of the body, and the holists, who see consciousness as the most personal evidence for a universal law – that the whole is more than the sum of the parts. What is the poor scientist to do when confronted with the rumour of a phenomenon, which is all that consciousness is? His

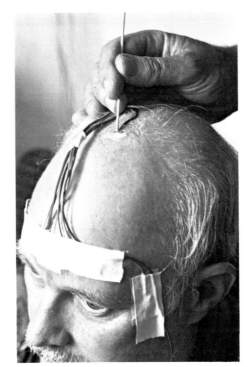

A volunteer is prepared for a night's sleep in Ian Oswald's laboratory at the University Department of Psychiatry in Edinburgh. The man has a cluster of electrodes stuck to his scalp and face to measure his eye movements and the electrical activity of his brain. While he sleeps these signals are constantly monitored on pen recorders. A tube running from a vein in his arm allows blood samples to be taken to assess the variation in hormone levels, etc., during sleep.

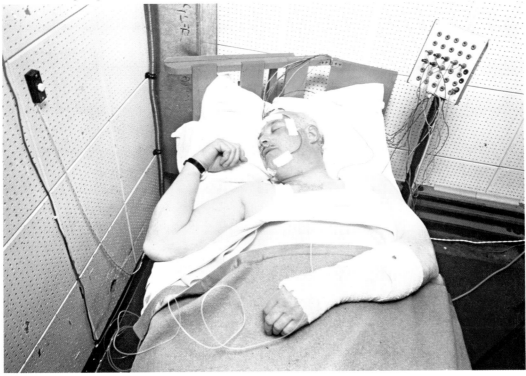

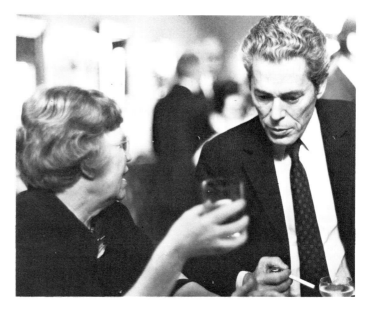

Jacques Monod (1910–1976) talking with anthropologist, Margaret Mead.

commitment to the 'postulate of objectivity', in the terminology of Jacques Monod, does not give the scientist methods to measure the private deliberation of the conscious mind.

How could a scientist deal with observations like these imaginary ones of Paul Jennings; 'When numbered pieces of toast and marmalade were dropped on various samples of carpet arranged in quality, from coir matting to the finest Kirman rugs, the marmalade-downwards incidence ($\mu\delta I$) varied indirectly with the quality of the carpet (Qc) – the Principle of the Graduated Hostility of Things.'

How can *Things* be hostile, the scientist must say. Faced with these improbable results, the physicist would surely conclude that some constituent in high-quality carpets exerts an attractive force, perhaps electrostatic or magnetic, on marmalade. The more cynical psychologist might suspect that the hostility was not in the toast itself but in the subtle intentions of the person who dropped it.

Most scientists are embarrassed when they cannot explain events by the forces and laws that they already

34

understand. Those who study the brain usually shuffle their feet uncomfortably and quickly change the subject when the discussion turns to that one brain function that we all know so intimately – consciousness itself. If *Things* cannot be hostile, how can the bits and pieces of molecular hardware that make up the brain have emotions and thoughts? The brain researcher of today is almost as impotent to evaluate consciousness as a computer is to judge beauty or put a price on a Rembrandt portrait. But it does not follow that beauty is *more* than the sum of a number of definable features, nor that a Rembrandt is *more* than all its individual brush strokes. The problem is to define all the brush strokes of the brain before we reject an opinion like that of W. Somerset Maugham, who said: 'The highest activities of consciousness have their origins in physical occurrences of the brain just as the loveliest melodies are not too sublime to be expressed by notes.'

There is no reason to believe that the scientific method will fail to account for the phenomenon of human consciousness, without invoking a new transcendent principle. Indeed, some would say that there is no *phenomenon* to explain.

In his remarkable book, *The Concept of Mind*, the Oxford philosopher Gilbert Ryle attempted to show that the everyday use of linguistic terms associated with the concept of consciousness, like 'believing' and 'thinking', is based on a logically untenable model of the mind as a 'Ghost in the Machine' – an independent, invisible and secret agent whose actions are intangible and cannot be revealed. Ryle rejected the doctrine that each of us is privy to an inner world of ghostly happenings, and gave an account of our lives as conscious beings in terms of *observable* actions and dispositions. Words like 'knowing' and 'believing' describe *propensities* to act in particular ways, under certain circumstances. If this kind of unmasking of consciousness destroys its special

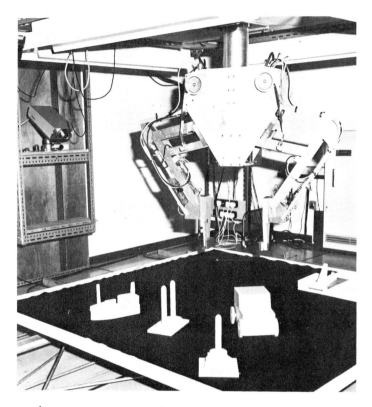

Could a computer be conscious? The study of artificial intelligence is an extremely active field at the moment; it is directed not only towards the design of more efficient machines, but also towards the understanding of human thought. 'Freddy', a robot at the Department of Machine Intelligence, Edinburgh, is operated by a large computer. His huge mechanical 'hand' can rotate and delicately handle small objects, like the toys that he is playing with here. The hand cannot move from side to side: instead the computer moves the large table, which constitutes Freddy's world. Freddy's sense organ is the camera viewing the table.

qualities, must we conclude that consciousness does not exist at all? To call 'knowing' a disposition to act may bring consciousness within the professional realm of brain research (and that is an important step), but it does not mean that there is nothing to explain. Ryle may have exorcised the Ghost from the Machine but he has left a Machine of much greater complexity.

Then is consciousness (as some reductionists insist) a mere epiphenomenon that results from the actions of an immensely complex but wholly mechanical brain? Such a view might imply that any complicated calculating machine would automatically be conscious. But few would claim that the world's combined telephone network, an undeniably enormous system of switches, has consciousness. Hostility, perhaps, but consciousness, surely not.

On the other hand, I am sure it is wrong to believe

that no computing machine can ever be conscious. But the property of awareness will not simply emerge at some mystical threshold of complexity. Those features that will give a computer consciousness will probably have to be designed into it just as deliberately as it is told how to multiply or divide. In fact, a conscious computer might actually be a better computer for the kind of tasks that we do well; it might even *enjoy* winning a game of chess!

The first requirement of a conscious machine (though perhaps not a guarantee of consciousness) is *motivation*. The nervous system did not first evolve as a device for intellectual exercise and conscious reflection; it simply made animals better at achieving their biological goals of eating, drinking and reproducing themselves – things that do not interest most computers!

If evolution has given us internal awareness, it must presumably have had survival value. One advantage that consciousness provides us is the ability to make predictions about the behaviour of *other* people, or even of other animals. It supplies a set of rules for relating emotional states to external events, which must surely be valuable in the complex social intercourse that governs the lives of people, no less than of chimpanzees or of the wild dogs of Africa.

When asked by the hostess at a rather boring party whether he was enjoying himself, Oscar Wilde is reputed to have replied that he certainly was, for there was no one else there to enjoy! And in his play, *An Ideal Husband*, Wilde wrote: 'Other people are quite dreadful. The only possible society is oneself.' But in a society of one, consciousness might not be needed at all.

Nothing illustrates better the need for society in the creation of consciousness than a remarkable experiment of Ronald Melzack. He reared some dogs in total isolation, from infancy to maturity, so that they had no opportunity to learn the rules of social interaction.

Darwin made fascinating observations on the expression of emotion in animals and man, and was interested in the biological continuity of the underlying mechanisms. He believed that contrasting emotions, like rage and affection, were demonstrated by opposite postures and signals. The snarl of a dog and the display of an enraged cat consist of a set of signals almost exactly the opposite of those used to convey conciliation and subservience.

37

When he released the dogs and studied their behaviour, he discovered that they seemed to have little or no sense of pain, or at least nothing more than a brief reflex response to it. They would return again and again to sniff at a burning match, and were quite unable to learn the danger of it.

And in his famous work on conditioned reflexes, Ivan Pavlov was even able to transform overt pain to apparent pleasure. In one experiment, instead of combining a ringing bell with morsels of food to teach a dog to salivate to a neutral stimulus, Pavlov used a brief electrical shock to the dog's paw as the 'unconditioned' signal that food was about to appear. Now at first the dog reacted violently to each shock and its appetite was decidedly reduced. But gradually a surprising transformation took place. The electric shock no longer prompted any sign of pain. On the contrary, when the shock came, the dog salivated, wagged its tail, and turned expectantly to its food bowl.

Philosophers from Aristotle to Ludwig Wittgenstein, from René Descartes to Peter Singer (the author of a recent book entitled *Animal Liberation*), have argued that the *expressions* of emotion and thought are the means by which each human or animal communicates its consciousness. For Descartes, animals had no rational soul; they could not verbalize propositional thoughts in

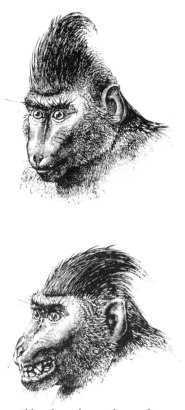

Although monkeys and apes often bare their teeth as a sign of anger, Darwin believed that a less exaggerated expression indicated pleasure and that this was the homologue of the human smile. Here a Celebes black ape (Cynopithecus niger) is shown in a placid state (above) and during the pleasure of being caressed (below).

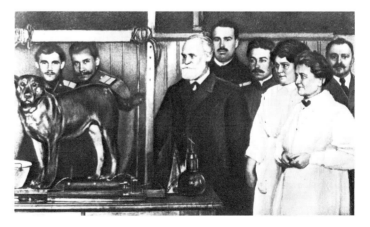

Ivan Pavlov (bearded) demonstrating to students at the Russian Army Medical Academy, in about 1904. Though Pavlov (1849–1936) is best known for his work on 'conditioned' reflexes, he won the Nobel Prize in 1904 for his earlier work on the physiology of digestion.

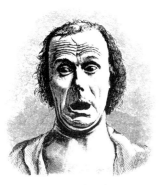

Terror, Darwin thought, is expressed by contraction of the sheet of muscle that stretches over the neck and chest. Sir Charles Bell called this the 'muscle of fright'. The mouth is pulled open with the lips drawn back, and at the same time the eyes start from their sockets. Here the expression was synthesized in a man, by electrical stimulation of the muscles through electrodes placed on his skin.

speech and were therefore not conscious. But Singer reasons that feelings, principally those produced by pain, can be ascribed to others, including animals, by observing reliable behavioural signs that we recognize as similar to the responses we ourselves produce when we consciously experience pain. What then are we to make of the observations of Melzack and Pavlov, which seem to show that the emotional state of pain is not related in a simple way to a particular stimulus? Behaviour, the overt product of consciousness, is modified by social as well as personal experience.

In man, too, cultural factors are extremely important in setting not only the threshold but also the context of pain. Religious martyrs could experience ecstasy rather than agony as they were tortured to death, and equally, some unfortunate people develop the severest pain with no apparent organic cause whatsoever. In the West, childbirth is often considered to be a dreadfully painful and potentially dangerous experience; but in some cultures it is the father, not the mother, who appears to suffer intensely as the child is born, even to the extent of his staying in bed with the baby to recover while his wife returns to the fields to work.

Acupuncture, itself unpleasant in the eyes of most Westerners, has been practised for more than two thousand years in China for the treatment of organic illness, and is, since the Cultural Revolution, quite often employed as the only form of anaesthetic in certain major surgical operations. Children in China are taught the classical theories and even the techniques of acupuncture from an early age and some would argue that the undeniable success of acupuncture analgesia amongst the Chinese is simply due to a kind of cultural conditioning, like that of Pavlov's dogs.

Yet it is possible that acupuncture analgesia, and perhaps other cultural modifiers of pain, operate through a simple physiological principle. It has been known for

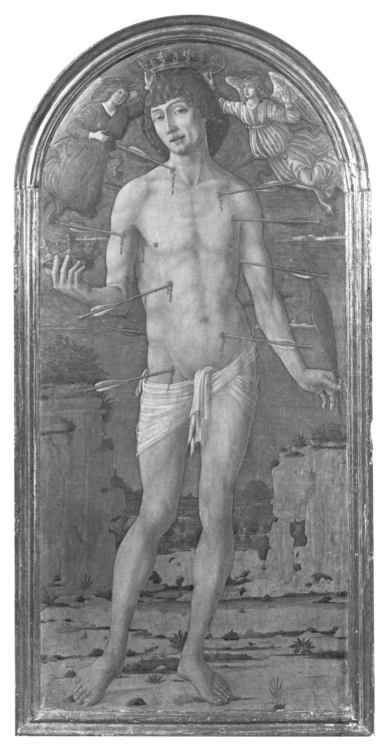

The cultural context of pain. 'St Sebastian' by Matteo di Giovanni (1435–1495). The National Gallery, London.

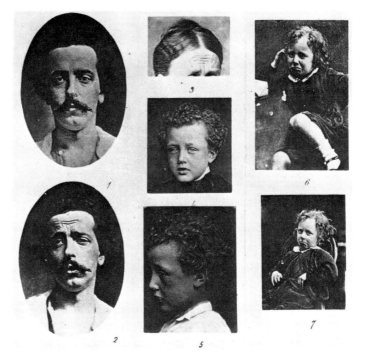

Darwin made a careful study of human facial expression and particularly of what he believed is a specific response to grief. The forehead is thrown into furrows and the eyebrows become oblique, with their inner ends drawn up. He found that few people could make this expression voluntarily: photograph 1 shows the relaxed expression and 2 the grieved expression of a young man; 3 shows the grief furrows on the forehead of a woman. The boy, whose normal face appears in 4, was photographed with oblique eyebrows, in 5, just before he burst into tears. People in low spirits, especially children, often have turned-down corners of the mouth (6 and 7).

many years that the pain-killing drug morphine and its derivatives act by attaching themselves to neurons in the brain – cells that somehow influence the threshold and sensation of pain. A naturally occurring substance named *enkephalin*, a tiny peptide molecule, has now been discovered in the brain; it acts just like morphine and reduces pain. In fact, it is presumably more accurate to say that morphine, the external agent, works just like enkephalin, the internal one. Enkephalin is a 'natural opiate', an analgesic drug that the brain itself can apparently synthesize to alleviate its own sensation of pain. Now Chinese scientists have recently reported that the practice of acupuncture on a rabbit causes the production of a substance in its brain which, when injected into the brain of another rabbit, increases its tolerance of discomfort. This substance might well be enkephalin, secreted by nerve cells in the brain in response to the acupuncture needles.

Morphine and the related compound heroin are dan-

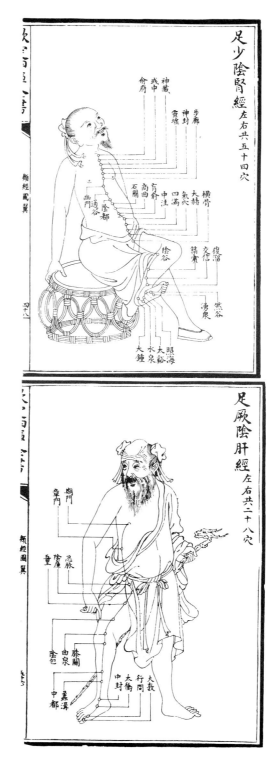

According to Lu Gwei-Djen and Joseph Needham (1978), acupuncture may have originated in the lancing of abscesses with sharp splinters of stone. After the discovery of iron and the manufacture of steel, metal needles were used, and a complex system of treatment of disease grew up in ancient China. It was based on the idea that blood and vital energy circulate in channels ('jing') in the body. The channels were plotted out as 'meridians' or 'tracts' on the skin, each relating to a particular group of deep organs; insertion and manipulation of needles at special 'points' along these tracts was thought to re-establish the balance of 'yin' and 'yang', upset by disease of any organ.

The Chinese now place less emphasis on the concept of channels, though they are continuing research in an attempt to prove their existence and physical structure. These two illustrations are from the Imperial Edition (1782) of the Lei Ching (1624), by Chang Chieh-Pin. Above is the reno-seminal tract with fifty-four acu-points: below is the liver tract with twenty-eight points.

42

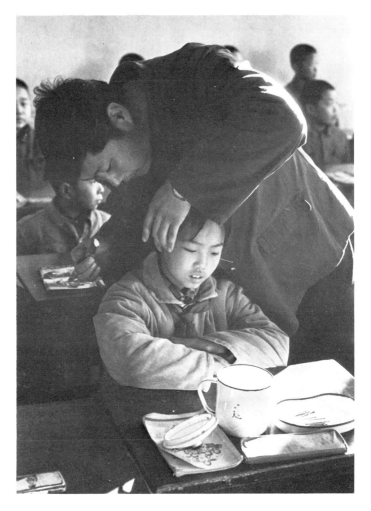

Children in a school for deaf-mutes in Peking are treated by acupuncture. New points are still being added to the classical schemes and many of them are around the ear. Here the medical worker holds a match to warm the needle (moxibustion). The Chinese claim modest success in the treatment of such children.

gerously addictive drugs and their unsupervised possession is illegal; yet we may all carry within our heads a 'natural opiate' that our brains use to regulate this most fundamental aspect of consciousness, the perception of pain.

For scientific, as well as philosophical, debate it is important to distinguish the *state* of consciousness from the so-called *actions* of the conscious mind, like choosing, whose existence as genuine operations Ryle and others would deny. It is this active aspect of consciousness that still gives scientists nightmares, philosophers headaches and theologians eternal joy. The question of *choice* is often the subject of acrimonious debate between reductionists and theists; so it is curious to hear arguments from both sides of the fence that the actions of man are entirely predetermined, either by the totally predictable and mechanical operations of the connections in his brain or by the predestination written for us all in the diary of an equally mechanical god. This attitude, whatever the motivation behind it, is an insult, either to the subtlety of the brain or to the mentality of God.

However, I see no reason why the alternative concept – choice of action – should necessarily be the exclusive property of those who believe in a permissive and forgiving deity. Some degree of flexibility of operation is the hallmark of an advanced machine. A robot that could calculate not only the apparently most favourable course of action or interpretation of events, but also other alternatives, and could try them all in turn, would have more chance of discovering successful strategies than one that invariably acted on what seemed to be the best decision. It is the serendipity of free will that makes it valuable.

Anyone who has tried to train an animal in a laboratory (or a child at home) knows that learning is never automatic nor totally predictable. It is a source of frustration to the behavioural psychologist that however well he trains a rat to run a maze, however easy the problem, the rat will never go in the correct direction on every single test. Now and then he exercises his ratty free will and takes the alley with no cheese at the end. But the choice that the psychologist calls incorrect is, for the rat, a potentially valuable paradigm of action – the chance to discover by chance the unexpected. By this analogy I do not mean to suggest that rats have conscious free will like man, nor to say that man is just a jumped-up rat, but it does illustrate that the existence of choice is not necessarily incompatible with a mechanical view of the mind. Just as one value of consciousness is to explain the

René Descartes had a typically hydraulic model of sleep. These cross-sections of the head, from Traité de l'Homme *(1664), show the pineal gland (H) sitting in the cavernous ventricle (E) under a mantle of whipped-cream – the cerebral hemispheres. In the upper drawing the brain is asleep; the production of animal spirit from the pineal gland has fallen to a trickle, so the ventricle has collapsed to a flabby bag and the nerve filaments (B) leading from it hang limply. In turn the muscles are relaxed. In the lower diagram the brain is awake, the spirit flowing, the nerves taut and muscles tense. It is interesting to compare this notion of a nervous system activated by central secretion of spirit with the modern concept of the reticular 'activating' system.*

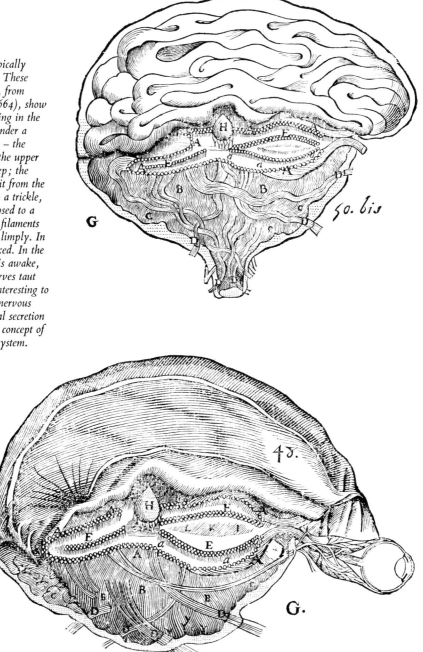

actions and emotions of others, the element of free will in conscious thought is an internal explanation for the flexibility of our *own* behaviour.

The final aspect of conscious experience, its level or state, is the one that can most readily be judged by objective observation; it can clearly be ascribed to animals and hence is most accessible to the scientific method. And that is why so much effort has been spent in the study of sleep.

The mysterious nature of sleep, and the dreams that it harbours, must always have occupied the thoughts of men. In the egg-shaped universe of Greek mythology, Night, the shell of the egg, gave birth to Hypnos, god of sleep, whose son was Morpheus, god of dreams, master of the fantasy land that lay close to the realm of the dead. There was widespread belief in the ancient world that sleep was a time of communication with the gods, a time when the spirit left the body to wander alone; and its experiences were the dreams of the night. The Egyptians slept on wooden pillows carved with the image of Bes, the god of highways, to protect the spirit on its night-time journey. And the ancient Chinese would never rouse a sleeper hastily, in case his spirit did not have time to re-enter his body. The view that we lose our personality in sleep is still prevalent. Even the Law seems to accept that a man is not responsible for his actions while asleep: courts in both the United States and Great Britain have acquitted people of murder when the act was committed during sleep. Curiously, the Law finds it less easy to forgive a man for *failing* to act because he falls asleep; a train driver in Yugoslavia was recently jailed for 15 years for sleeping at the controls of a train that crashed at Zagreb in 1974, killing 153 people.

It is probably the apparent futility of sleep, the wasted time, the biological danger of it, that leads us to cherish dreams, the sole conscious product of sleep. The inter-

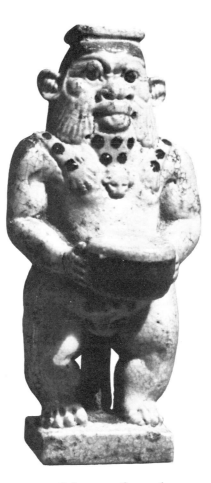

Faience figure of Bes, the god of highways who protected the travelling spirit of the sleeper (c. 1300 B.C.).

preters of dreams, from the second-century sooth-sayer Artemidorus of Ephesus to Sigmund Freud, have capitalized on our fascination with these products of the unbridled mind.

But the similarity between the untrustworthy image of the dream and waking experience has posed enormous problems for the philosopher. The Chinese Taoist, Chuang Tzu, in the third century B.C., was one of the first to express his fears. He wrote of himself: 'Once upon a time, I, Chuang Tzu, dreamed I was a butterfly flying happily here and there . . . suddenly I woke up and I was indeed Chuang Tzu. Did Chuang Tzu dream he was a butterfly, or did the butterfly dream he was Chuang Tzu?

47

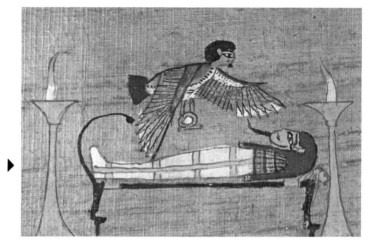

Sleep and death were thought of as times when the soul left the body to wander alone. 'The Ba Spirit over the Mummy', from the papyrus of Ani, Theban Book of the Dead, Egypt (C. 1250 B.C.).

Jacob's dream of the ladder with angels ascending and descending. Judaism and Christianity both emphasized the dream as a medium of communication with heaven. From an early fourteenth-century French manuscript (MS Douce 211, f 30), Bodleian Library, Oxford).

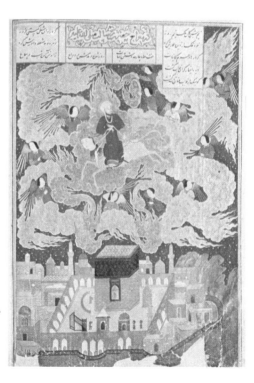

Mohammed's dream, the 'Lailatal-Miraj' or 'Night Journey': he rides over Kaba on Elboraq (half man, half silver mare). Persian miniature from the Khamsa of Nizami, 1494.

48

In most religions, dreams are incidents of mystical insight, of communion with the gods and of divine revelation. The Bible is full of dreams, from Jacob's ladder and Joseph's wheat sheaves to the premonitions of Pontius Pilate's wife. In his great dream of initiation, Mohammed was given the silver horse Elboraq, which he rode to Jerusalem and then on through all the spheres of celestial existence to God himself.

The irrational view that dreams are veiled predictions of future events was, and still is, widely held. The analytical psychologist Erich Fromm has tried to justify this belief by arguing that, if dreams are, as Freud suggested, the disguised fulfilment of unconscious wishes, then they might be expected to portray episodes that will be unwittingly sought out in real life. Aristotle, two thousand years ago, took a more jaundiced view, saying that since dreams come in such abundance and such variety, some of them will inevitably resemble future events, just by chance – perhaps the first example of a statistical argument in the behavioural sciences!

However, it was a belief in the power of premonition and even the existence of telepathic communication that led to the single most important technical advance in the study of sleep, the measurement of the human electro-encephalogram or EEG. Towards the end of the last century, a young German, Hans Berger, who was serving in the army, slipped from his horse as it stumbled down an embankment, and he narrowly escaped serious injury. That evening he was astonished to receive a telegram from his father asking if he was well, because his sister had had a feeling that he was in danger.

This event led Berger to change his studies from astronomy to psychiatry at the University of Jena, where he received his doctorate in 1897, just at the time that Sigmund Freud was writing *The Interpretation of Dreams* in Vienna. Berger was obsessed with the relationship between material events in the brain and mental

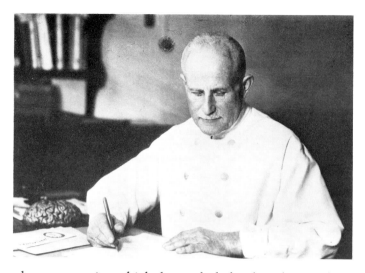

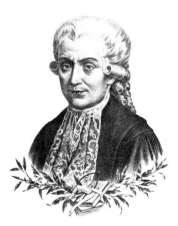

Hans (Johannes) Berger (1873–1941).

Luigi Galvani (1737–1798).

phenomena, in which he included telepathy. A long tradition of experiments, started by John Walsh in England and Luigi Galvani in Italy, has established that signals are carried along nerves to muscles in the form of electrical pulses. It was known that the brain is packed with nerve cells and fibres, and electrical activity had already been detected in the brains of animals. Berger hoped to prove that electrical responses in the brains of men are correlated with consciousness and might even be the physical medium by which thoughts could be telepathically transmitted. He was using hopelessly in-sensitive electronic equipment and at first was frustrated by failure, but in 1924 he managed to record a signal with metal electrodes stuck to the head of his young son Klaus.

But what strange signals they were! Whenever Klaus was relaxed and inattentive, Berger picked up a feeble but definite ripple of electrical potential, with a regular frequency of about 10 cycles each second: he called it the *alpha rhythm*. Much more exciting, Berger later found that these electrical waves of the brain certainly were influenced by conscious experience. He wrote: 'In many experimental subjects, opening of the eyes ... caused an immediate change in the EEG and ... during

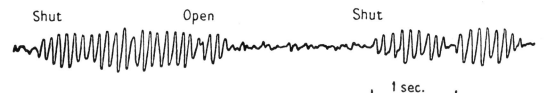

Shut   Open   Shut

1 sec.

Edgar, Lord Adrian, then Professor of Physiology in Cambridge, did a great deal in the 1930s to bring Berger's findings to the attention of the initially-sceptical scientific community. Adrian confirmed, and enlarged on, many of Berger's discoveries. This EEG recording of Adrian and Matthews (1934) shows Adrian's own alpha rhythm welling up each time he closed his eyes and desynchronizing as he opened them. Adrian found that the rhythm was strongest over the back of the skull, above the visual area of the cerebral hemispheres, and that just 'thinking about', and attending to, a spot of light in the peripheral visual field can break up the alpha rhythm.

mental tasks, e.g. when solving a problem of arithmetic, the mere naming of the task sometimes caused the same change.' It was something of a disappointment to Hans Berger, however, that this change that occurred in the EEG when a person became more alert was not an increase in the amplitude of his alpha rhythm, but its virtual disappearance. The EEG became *desynchronized* and decomposed into a torrent of tiny high frequency waves. But at least Berger had shown that the human brain, no less than that of an animal, is electrically active and that alterations in mood, attention and the state of consciousness are accompanied by (some would say caused by) modulations of the electrical rhythm. Though we still do not know the exact origin of this rhythm, it does seem to relate to the chatter of impulses in the nerve cells of the great cerebral cortex – the convoluted mantle that enwraps the whole brain and is so richly developed in man.

During the delicious drowsiness that heralds sleep, the alpha rhythm dominates; as sleep deepens, the waves of the EEG become longer and slower in frequency. This mindless rhythm is, in a sense, the natural state of the brain; it is the pattern adopted when sensory stimulation is attenuated and vigilance is low. Indeed some classical experiments between 1930 and 1950 suggested that sleep is essentially a passive affair. A large, untidy tangle of nerve cells and fibres, called the *reticular formation*, in the stem of the brain, was implicated in the maintenance of consciousness. Like a great computer without a power supply, the cerebral cortex without the reticular formation below it is only a potentially powerful machine. Damage to the reticular formation can produce a pro-

51

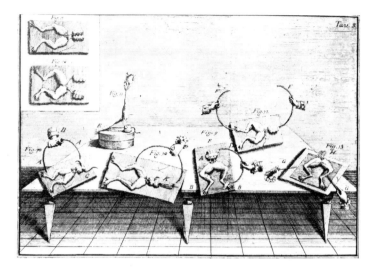

longed state of coma and unconsciousness, and brief electrical stimulation of it in animals will rudely awaken them from sleep and abolish the lazy rhythms from their EEG.

Many sensory nerve fibres, bringing information into the brain from the sense organs, have branches that terminate in the reticular formation, in addition to their main trunk lines that run up towards the cerebral cortex. Any incoming signal is thought to have two effects: first to inform a particular part of the cortex about the nature of the new event, and second to activate the connections between the reticular formation and the whole cortex, hence desynchronizing its waves.

But the relentless daily demand for sleep, the internal clock that would not let Nathaniel Kleitman adopt the schedule of a different world, and the infinite torment of struggling to resist the embraces of Hypnos, all demonstrate that sleeping and waking are not passive reflections of sensory input. Indeed, regular gentle electrical stimulation in many parts of the brain, including the lowest parts of the reticular formation itself, can throw the cortical EEG of an alert cat into rhythmic waves, and the cat will instantly settle down and drift into completely normal sleep. More than sixty years ago two French-

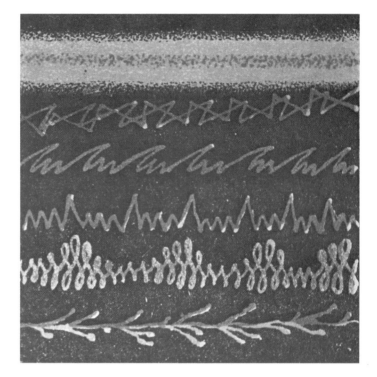

In 1867 Marquis d'Hervey de Saint-Denis made this strange picture (almost like an EEG recording) of his own 'hypnagogic' visions seen as he drifted off to sleep. He described them as 'bright lines that cross and interlace, that roll up and make circles, lozenges and other geometric shapes'.

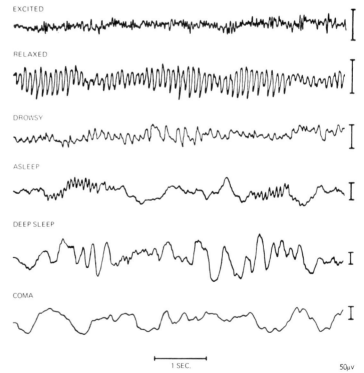

EXCITED

RELAXED

DROWSY

ASLEEP

DEEP SLEEP

COMA

1 SEC.

50µv

Typical EEG recordings, showing the change from high-frequency, low-amplitude waves during excitement, through the alpha rhythm of relaxation, to the very large, low-frequency waves of sleep or coma. Paradoxical sleep is not shown in these records. (Results of H. H. Jasper, 1941. The vertical markers on the right all indicate a voltage of just 50 microvolts.)

53

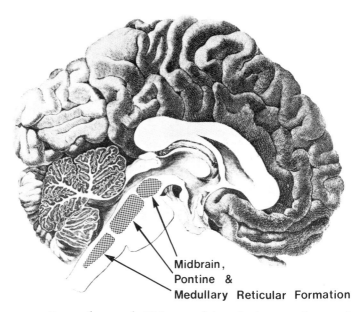

The midbrain reticular formation, thought to be involved in maintaining the arousal of the cerebral hemispheres, is shown, together with the medullary and pontine areas that may play a part in the active control of the cycles of slow-wave sleep and paradoxical sleep. The illustration itself, which shows an inside view of the left half of the human brain, is from a book published in 1796 by the excellent anatomist, Samuel Soemmerring (1755–1830).

Midbrain,
Pontine &
Medullary Reticular Formation

men, Legendre and Piéron, claimed that a chemical substance builds up in the brain of a tired animal and that if the fluid from the ventricles is transfused into those of another animal, the latter will fall asleep. This unlikely story has now been all but proved by John Pappenheimer and his colleagues at Harvard Medical School. A substance, factor S, isolated from the cerebral fluid of sleepy goats, will greatly enhance the sleep of rats or rabbits into whose brain it is transfused. It seems likely that factor S is, like enkephalin, a small peptide molecule, which gradually builds up during the waking period and possibly acts on brain stem regions that trigger the start of sleep.

Finally, measurement of the EEG has thrown light on the mystery of dreams themselves. In 1952 two students in Kleitman's laboratory, Eugene Aserinsky and William Dement, discovered that at roughly ninety-minute intervals throughout the night extraordinary things happened on the recording machine attached to their sleeping volunteers. The EEG suddenly reverted to the drowsy mode, as if the sleeper were about to wake up; his breathing became irregular, his heart rate increased, his fingers twitched and, if the volunteer was male, his penis sprang to attention. Most striking of all, his eyes beneath their lids darted about crazily. These episodes are therefore called rapid-eye movement sleep, or paradoxical sleep, because the sleeper is actually harder to awaken despite his more alert EEG. Dement went on to find that if someone *is* woken in this stage of sleep, he is almost certain to say that he had just had a vivid dream. Moreover, if someone is selectively deprived of just paradoxical sleep, by being woken each time it starts, he is (perhaps not surprisingly) slightly irritable during the following day, and the next night he spends much more time than usual in paradoxical sleep – conceivably catching up on his need to dream.

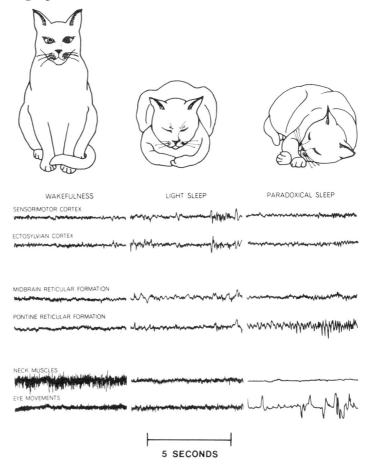

These records were made by Michel Jouvet, who has studied intensively the regulation of normal (light) sleep and paradoxical sleep in cats. The first two traces show the EEG recorded from different parts of the cerebral hemisphere: the large waves seen during light sleep are absent during waking and paradoxical sleep. The same pattern is seen in the midbrain (activating) reticular formation, but the pontine reticular formation is rhythmically active during paradoxical sleep (it is thought to set off some of the unexpected events of this very deep stage of sleep, such as the large, jerky eye movements). In cats, the most distinctive feature of paradoxical sleep is the sudden relaxation of body muscles especially those of the neck, causing the cat's characteristic posture.

WAKEFULNESS   LIGHT SLEEP   PARADOXICAL SLEEP

SENSORIMOTOR CORTEX

ECTOSYLVIAN CORTEX

MIDBRAIN RETICULAR FORMATION

PONTINE RETICULAR FORMATION

NECK MUSCLES

EYE MOVEMENTS

5 SECONDS

Kleitman and his student, William Dement, discovered the regular appearance of pardoxical sleep, about every ninety minutes during the night. They classified the depth of normal sleep into four stages, depending on the amplitude of low-frequency waves. The depth of sleep swings up and down, with fairly regular episodes of paradoxical sleep (P), each lasting about twenty minutes. The EEG returns to a relatively desynchronized state and the eyes jerk back and forth from time to time. Kleitman thought that this periodicity within sleep represents an inherent rhythm of activity, every sixty to ninety minutes, that is most clearly seen in the sleep cycles of newborn babies. Many experimenters have reported that adults, even when awake, have periods of slightly increased body movement, and a greater tendency to eat, drink or smoke, approximately every ninety minutes.

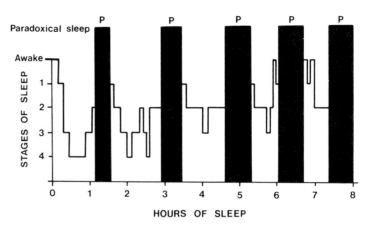

Neurons usually communicate with each other by means of chemical 'transmitter substances', produced by the terminals of nerve fibres at their points of contact with other nerve cells. (This process is described in more detail in Chapter 3). This photomicrograph, prepared by Barry Everitt, is of a thin section of the brain stem of a rat, which has been chemically treated to make certain transmitter substances fluorescent, and therefore luminous under ultraviolet illumination. One bundle of nerve fibres (upper right) contains the transmitter noradrenaline, and the mass of cell bodies and fibres (lower half) contains 5-hydroxy-tryptamine. Some of the neurons producing these two transmitter substances send their fibres up to the cerebral cortex, and they may be involved in the regulation of normal and paradoxical sleep.

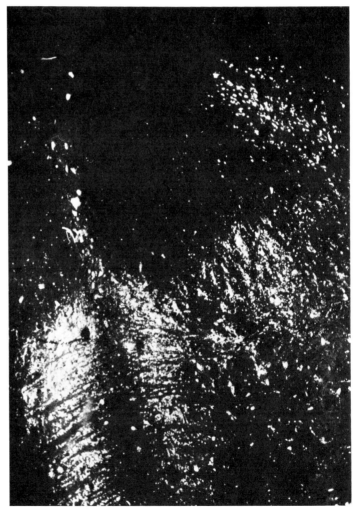

Now experiments with animals point to another area in the brain stem reticular formation as the site of initiation of paradoxical sleep. This region may activate the cerebral cortex and trigger the spurious mental events of dreams. But at the same time an almost total inhibition occurs at the level of the spinal cord, so that the muscles of the body are not thrown into seizures by the violent activity of the brain. Only the movements of fingers, eyes, and so on, escape this paralysis.

The level of consciousness is then regulated by a primitive part of the brain, not by the intellectual machinery of the cerebral cortex. This raises ethical and legal dilemmas of the most serious kind. The rapid advances in heart transplantation surgery a few years ago played a part in changing the public and legal attitude to dying. The present medical definition of death accepts the fact that a man, as an independent mind, can outlive his own heart. As in the recent case of Karen Quinlan in the United States, death is now equated with irreparable damage to the brain stem, even when the higher centres

'Landscape from a Dream', 1936–1938, by Paul Nash.

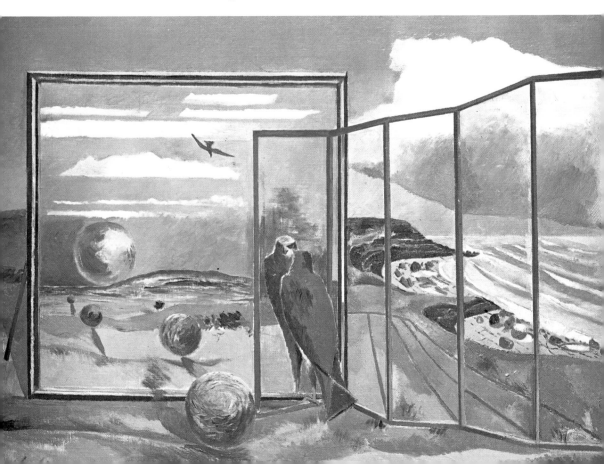

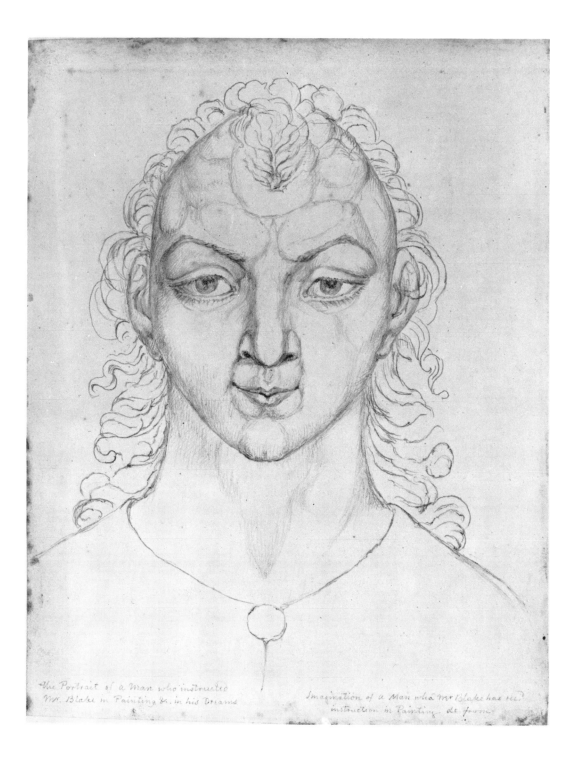

The Portrait of a Man who instructed
Mr. Blake in Painting &c. in his Dreams

Imagination of a Man who Mr Blake has rec.d
instruction in Painting &c from

of the cerebral cortex are quite intact. Without the vital power that drives it, the mind may be suspended forever in sleep. But it would be short-sighted to think that this interpretation is less expedient and more absolute than one based on the function of the heart. Even our definition of life itself is determined by the prevailing level of medical expertise and current scientific opinion. If for no other reason, the experimental study of sleep is important; a full understanding of the control of consciousness may give us more objective criteria for the definition of death.

◀

'The Portrait of a Man who instructed Mr Blake in Painting and in his Dreams'. Copy (c. 1819), by John Linnell, of a pencil drawing by William Blake.

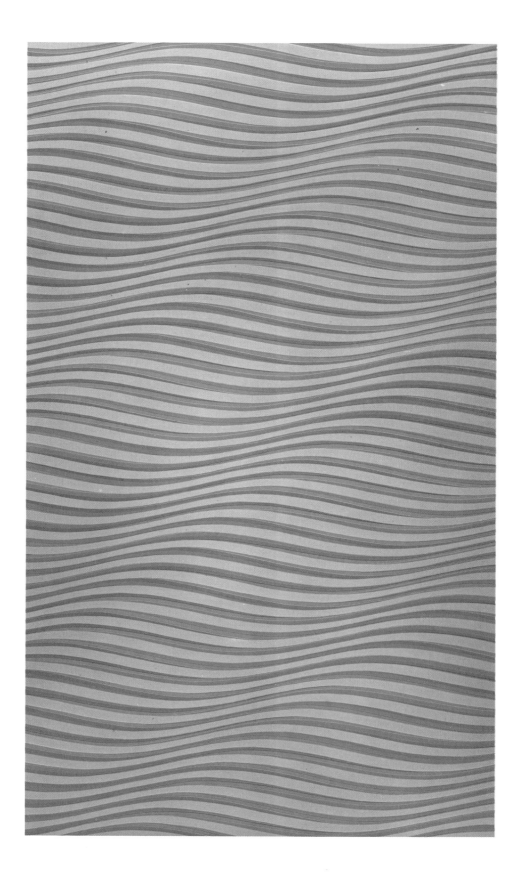

3 An image of truth

Rien ne m'est seur que la chose incertaine:
Obscur, fors ce qui est tout evident;
Doubte, ne fais, fors en chose certaine;
Science tiens a soudain accident,
Je gaigne tout et demeure perdent;
Au point du jour dis: 'Dieu vous doint bon soir!'
Gisant envers, j'ay grant paour de cheoir;
J'ay bien de quoy et si n'en ay pas ung;

I put all my trust in things that I doubt:
The obvious alone is unclear;
Certainty never knows what it's about,
And truth from sheer chance will appear.
I'm still just a loser although I win all;
'Good night' I say at day's dawning.
Even in bed I'm scared that I'll fall;
And I've only got plenty of nothing.

François Villon (1431–c. 1465), *Ballade*

In Cambridge, Massachusetts, in London, England, and in Lyon, France, there are men who can see but do not perceive. They have eyes that function, but they themselves are unaware of the things that their eyes can see and on which they are able to act. These men all have brain injuries at the back of the cerebral hemispheres, in the part called the visual cortex, which receives messages from the eyes.

In the middle of the last century, a Frenchman, Marie-Jean-Pierre Flourens, provided the first real experimental

Gouache on paper, 1976, by Bridget Riley.

61

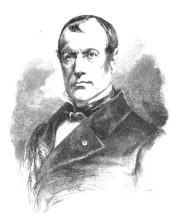

Marie-Jean-Pierre Flourens (1794–1867).

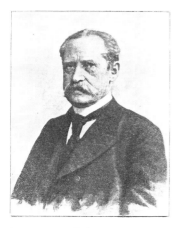

Hermann Munk (1839–1912).

evidence that the cerebral cortex is responsible for so-called 'higher functions' of the mind. Although he spoke of faculties like will and intellect, his experimental subjects were animals, not people. Like Aristotle, Galen and Leonardo before him, Flourens had intuitive trust in the continuity of biological mechanisms, which led him to extrapolate from animals to man. Shortly before his death in 1867, Flourens wrote in opposition to Darwin's new theory of Natural Selection, but it was that very theory that made legitimate his own experimental paradigm. Flourens worked by studying the consequences on an animal's behaviour of damage to its brain.

'Animals deprived of their cerebral lobes,' he concluded, 'have . . . neither perception, nor judgement, nor memory, nor will. . . . The cerebral lobes are therefore the exclusive seat of all the perceptions and all the intellectual faculties.'

He did not, however, believe that these various functions were *localized* in different parts of the cerebral hemispheres; but his methods were imprecise and in any case most of his observations were on birds, whose hemispheres are quite unlike those of a mammal.

Hermann Munk, in Berlin, first realized that small injuries to the surface of the cortex could render an animal apparently blind or seemingly deaf. But Munk also made the remarkable discovery that these 'mind-blind' and 'mind-deaf' animals quite rapidly recovered their senses; he likened their progress to young animals learning to appreciate their sensations for the first time.

How different the situation seemed to be when neurologists first turned their attention to the human cortex. It is a sad fact that brain science, no less than engineering and technology, has reaped a rich harvest of knowledge from the tragedy of war: the effects of damage to the brain were first systematically recorded during the Russo–Japanese war of 1904. The methods of aseptic surgery and the treatment of shock were advancing rapidly; so

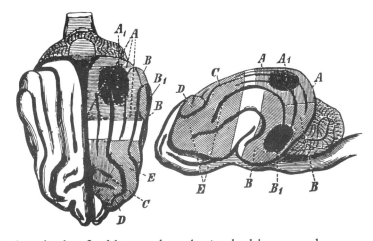

Hermann Munk's (1881) diagram of the dog's brain showing areas of the cerebral hemispheres where damage (on both sides) produced temporary 'mind-blindness' (A1) and 'mind-deafness' (B1). These regions lie within the visual and auditory receiving areas of the cortex.

hundreds of soldiers, whose brains had been on the trajectory of a splinter of shell or a fragment of shrapnel, survived and learned to use their injured minds. These precise brain wounds, often quite small, provide unique experiments of fate that allow us to compare ourselves with the animals of Flourens and Munk.

The First World War was a vast, unwanted experiment in neurology. In addition to the knowledge it gave of the 'shell shock' that men suffer when their minds are pushed to the limits of endurance, it added another catalogue of brain damage of the more overt kind. The Irish neurologist, Gordon Holmes, studied men whose injuries affected the posterior pole of the hemispheres, which Munk had implicated in the functions of seeing in animals. Holmes confirmed that a tiny area of damage here produced a corresponding patch of blindness, or *scotoma*, in the visual field. The patient stared fixedly at a point as Holmes mapped out the scotoma by waving a fine wand with a light on the end of it. Whenever the light fell into the affected part of the field it disappeared from the patient's view.

On the question of recovery of vision, however, Holmes' results were totally different from Munk's. The representation of the eyes in the visual cortex, he wrote, 'is fixed and immutable, so that if a part of the visual cortex be totally destroyed there will be a permanent

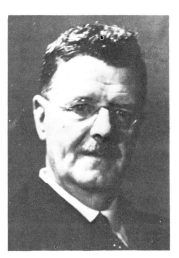

Sir Gordon Holmes (1876–1965).

63

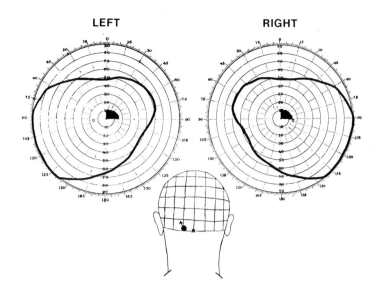

LEFT **RIGHT**

This is one of Holmes's original visual field maps. On 20 October 1916, a young private in the army was wounded by a fragment of shell-casing, which entered his skull at the point shown on the diagram of his head, travelling in the direction of the arrow. When tested ten days afterwards he was unaware of any defect in his vision. Nevertheless, careful mapping revealed a tiny patch of blindness, or scotoma, shown as a black area on each of the two maps of his visual field. (The field is shown separately for the left and right eyes.) The centre of each circular pattern shows the point of fixation of the eye. The pear-shaped outer line is the extreme edge of the visual field, which is quite normal in form. The scotoma lay just to the right and above the fixation point and was identical in shape in the two eyes. The brain injury was on the left side, showing that the visual cortex receives information from both eyes about the opposite half of the visual field.

blindness of the corresponding segment of the visual fields'. Holmes remeasured the blind areas years after the injury in some of his patients and found them quite unchanged.

But the new experiments, in the United States, England and France, show that such people can actually see without knowing it. The patients in question have in-dubitable injuries of the visual cortex; they never see a flashing light inside the resulting scotoma; in fact they deny seeing anything there at all. Yet if such a light is briefly flashed and they are asked to *guess* where it is by *pointing* to it, they do so with remarkable skill. They can even guess reliably whether a line flashed within the scotoma is horizontal or vertical, even though they claim that they see no line at all, and find the whole exercise rather foolish.

It is well known that some nerve fibres from the eyes send their signals to regions below the cerebral hemi-spheres, more primitive parts of the brain that are rather important in a frog, but were thought only to control movements of the eyes in man. Now we must accept that these sub-cortical visual areas are capable of pro-viding information for the movements of the hands and even for the guesses of an unaware mind. The phenomenon of 'blindsight', as it has been called, establishes that the cortex is the home of *conscious* perception, but some kind of sensory function can continue without it.

Then why, one might ask, have the cerebral cortex at all? What is it that the intact brain does that the man with 'blindsight' cannot do? It constructs a *description* of outside reality, a *model* in which it has confidence and sufficient faith to speak. According to the adage of William Blake: 'Every thing possible to be believed is an image of truth.' And what our perception provides us with is this 'image of truth', which we trust as a measure of reality. Between the turmoil of moving lights that fills the tiny image without our eye and the credible world of external *objects* that we build from that image is a miraculous transformation.

How easy it all was for some of the Greeks, most notably Euclid; light, he thought, streamed out from the eyes to touch the world, like a million invisible fingers. Objects were seen as objects because they were *felt* as solid and real by these seeing hands. The long fingers of vision certainly do free us from the tiny world within the reach of our arms. When Galileo became blind in 1638 he wrote: 'This heaven, this earth, this universe, which . . . I have enlarged a hundred, nay a thousand fold beyond the limits universally accepted by the learned men of all previous ages, are now shrivelled up for me into such a narrow compass as is filled by my own bodily sensations.'

But seeing is not like touching. An object held in the

The visual field plot of patient D.B., studied by Weiskrantz, Warrington, Sanders and Marshall (1974) in London. He had suffered from headaches and disturbances of vision since the age of fourteen and a malformation of blood vessels was detected over the right primary visual cortex. It was surgically removed in 1973 and he now has normal vision only in the area enclosed by the line on the right of the fixation point. By normal tests he is completely blind on his left side, except for a narrow crescent of partial vision in the upper left field (dotted area, enclosed by broken lines). He 'perceives' nothing that falls within the huge scotoma, but he can point with accuracy towards lights on the left side, and can even 'guess' whether a line flashed there is vertical or horizontal.

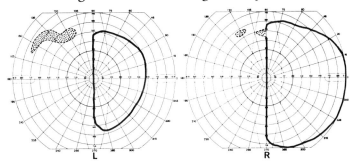

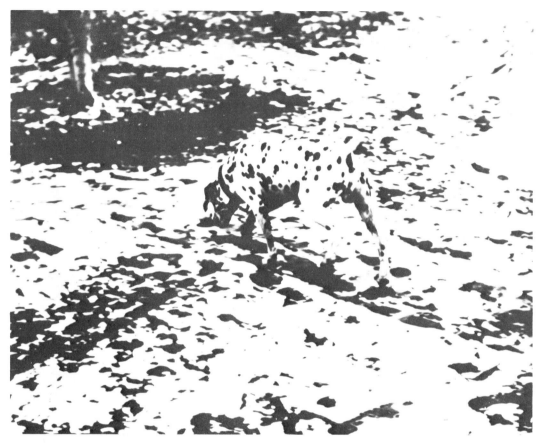

The ability to construct meaningful perceptual descriptions is quite remarkable. Organization is imposed on visual sensations; we struggle to see patterns as things, a process that fascinated Ludwig Wittgenstein. How do we manage to handle such fragmentary information as in this photograph by Ronald James?

hand is permanent, solid, immutable in size and shape: the patterns seen by the eyes change their size with their distance, and change their shape with their movement, as every artist knows. The fact is, of course, that the subjects of seeing are not objects themselves, but the flat, intangible images of them which hide within the pupil of the eye.

Light comes *into* the eye in a cone of straight rays, not *out* of it, as Euclid had said. The realization of this produced a revolution in Renaissance art, not just through the discovery of perspective, but because artists must have learned that their task was to challenge the viewer just as he is tested by the image in his own eye. The retina of the eye is the canvas of the brain. If we can conjure everything that we know of reality from the

66

poverty of its two-dimensional image, why should the artist not use his painting to provoke perceptions just as real? But to do so the painter who strives to represent reality must transcend his *own* perception. He must ignore or override the very mechanisms in his mind that create objects out of images. For we do not perceive our retinal *image*; we experience an externalized world of solid things.

In a way the Greeks were right. As you watch a man walk away, you see that he remains the same size (although the image of him on your retina certainly shrinks). Look at a coin when you turn it in your hands and you perceive it always as a round disc of metal (although its image is an infinite series of ellipses). What we reconstruct within the mind's eye are the *constant* physical properties of objects; and so we should, because those are the things that we *need* to know. To do this we

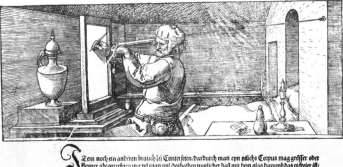

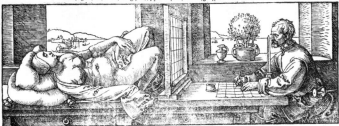

Light comes into the eye in a cone of straight rays. These woodcuts (c. 1527) by Albrecht Dürer show 'Leonardo's window', one of the methods used by artists to construct drawings in correct perspective, overcoming the constancy of their own perceptions.

67

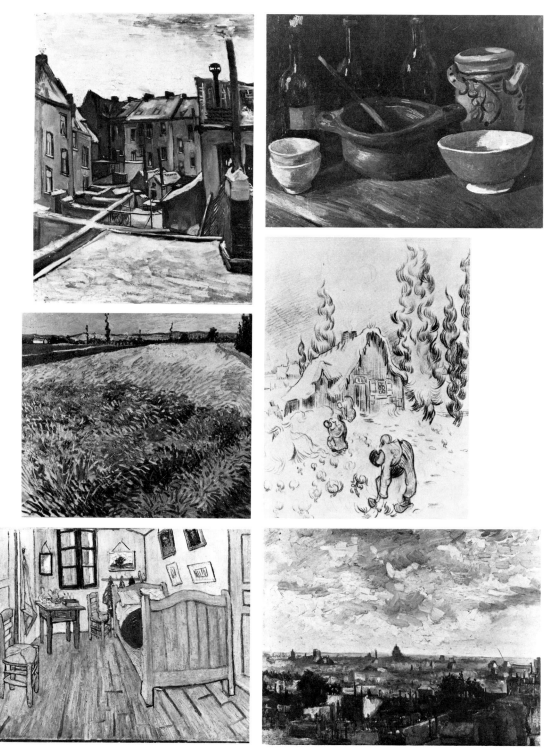

The artist, like the eye, must provide the clues of distance to tell his magic lies. Vincent Van Gogh (1853–1890) used all the artistic clues to distance distinctively in these six works.

First column, from top to bottom:
  Conventional linear perspective.
  The gradient of texture, becoming coarser in the foreground.
  The relative sizes of familiar objects.

Second column:
  Obscuring of distant objects by nearer ones.
  More distant objects are higher in the visual field.
  Decrease of contrast with distance.

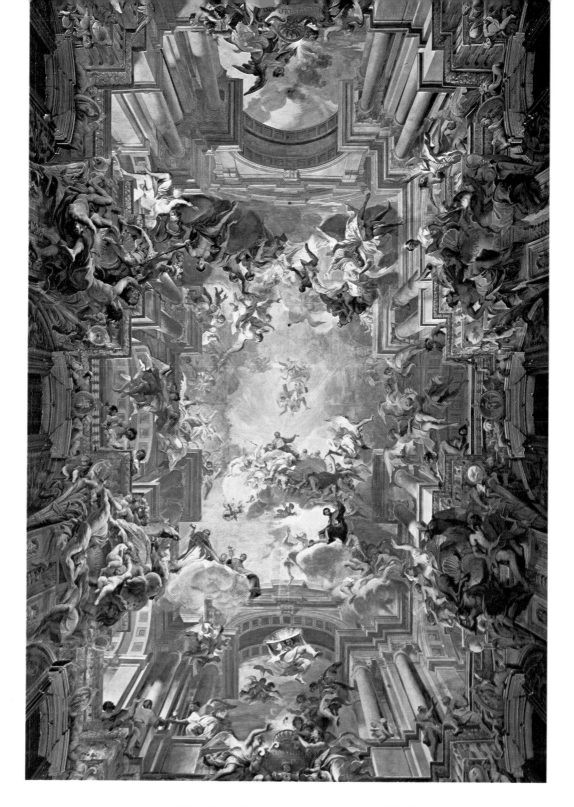

The ceiling of Sant' Ignazio in Rome, painted by Andrea Pozzo (1642–1709) between 1691 and 1694. The true surface of the ceiling is a smooth half–cylinder. Here it is viewed from a marble disc in the floor of the church, which marks the correct viewing point. Even Pozzo acknowledged the restrictive element in trompe l'oeil and he studied the deformation produced by viewing from other positions.

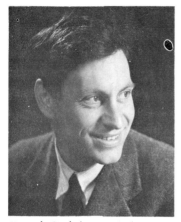

Kenneth Craik (1914–1945).

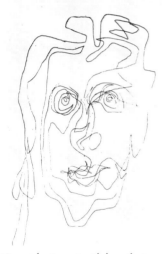

'I must begin, not with hypothesis, but with specific instances.' 'Altes Fraülein', 1931, by Paul Klee. © by SPADEM Paris, 1976.

must not only recognize the outlines of individual objects from the confusion within the eye, but must also discover from the image subtle clues about their distances. Only when we know both the true geometrical shapes in the image and the distances of the objects portrayed there can we derive the constancy of our perceptions. The artist, like the eye, must provide true images and the clues of distance to tell his magic lies.

The mechanisms of constant perception are built into our brains. They are either rapidly learned or they may even be inherited; a baby a few weeks old reacts as if his perceptions already have constancy of shape and size. The brilliant Cambridge psychologist, Kenneth Craik, who died tragically young in a road accident in 1945, was the first to argue strongly that perception is a model in the brain, a hypothesis about the world that presupposes the physical laws of movement and time. It took great minds like those of Isaac Newton and John Dalton to formulate the laws of motion and the conservation of matter in words and mathematics. But every child discovers a pictorial version of the physical laws of the universe in his own perceptions.

The representational artist, then, must be as perceptually naïve as an embryo; he must not illustrate his own model of the world but must search behind it for the image in his eye. As Paul Klee wrote in 1902: 'I must begin, not with hypothesis, but with specific instances, no matter how minute.'

Renaissance painters, starting with the pioneer of perspective, Filippo Brunelleschi, in the early fifteenth century, tried to create the *trompe l'oeil*, the deceit of the eye. Their greatest achievements are the extraordinary ceiling paintings, like those of Andrea Pozzo in the Church of Sant' Ignazio in Rome, where the artist has painted a continuation of the architecture of the building, soaring upwards and occupied by an unruly host of angels and cherubs with good heads for heights.

70

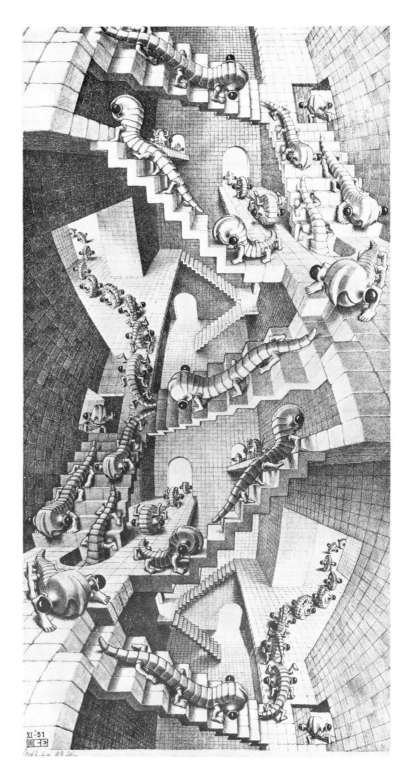

'House of stairs', 1951, by Maurits Escher (1898–1972). This painting is so disturbing, like many of the visual illusions, because there is no single internal model into which it can be fitted. One remarkable feature of paintings and drawings is that they can represent three-dimensional objects and scenes that are logically impossible in the real world.

71

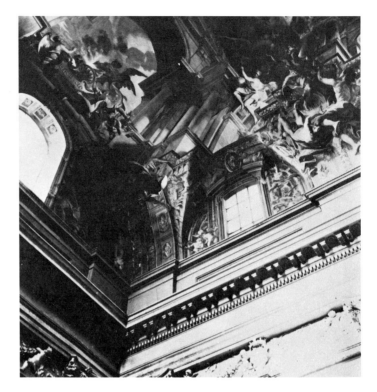

Here part of Pozzo's ceiling is photographed from an entirely wrong angle and the painted architecture, though still seen three-dimensionally, is grossly distorted, because the flat painting is interpreted as if it were a real solid object with its perspective centred on the inappropriate viewing point. This illustration is from Optics, Painting and Photography by M. H. Pirenne. Dr Pirenne, himself the son of a Belgian artist, Maurice Pirenne, was a pioneer in the application of the statistical principles of quantum physics to the question of the visibility of very dim lights. He has suggested that normal framed pictures are treated in a special way in our perceptions, because we recognize them as pictures by their frames or edges.

These ceiling paintings gain their magical transparency because they have no distinctive edge. There is nothing to identify them as paintings. But because a painting is nothing but a flat geometrical projection, its perspective can only be perfect from one viewing point. Only one observer in the church can see the painting as it should be seen. From any other position its geometry is wrong and its painted pillars and arches seem to twist and sag. Just when the artist succeeds in synthesizing exactly the retinal projection of an actual scene, then surely he fails, for he gives the privilege of perfection to one viewer alone.

Conventional paintings and drawings have a different and special quality. As the psychologist Richard Gregory has said: 'Pictures are paradoxes.' They are part of our actual world of objects and at the same time are messengers from a different world. We see them simultaneously as lines and colours on a flat surface and as the

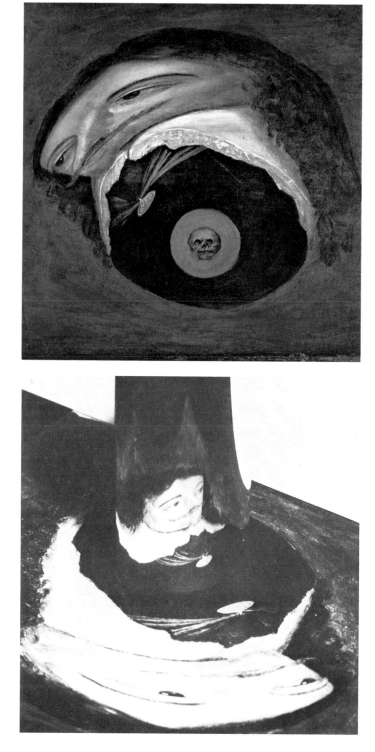

'Charles I of England', c. 1660, by an unknown artist. (National Portrait Gallery, Gripsholm, Sweden. 41 x 50 cm.) This extraordinary portrait is an example of anamorphosis – a distorted image that looks normal when viewed from a particular, unusual direction or through a distorting mirror. This example is seen correctly when reflected in a cylindrical mirror placed on the death's-head, as seen in the lower photograph. Anamorphosis started with the realization that any picture drawn in exact perspective is only correctly seen from a single viewing point – straight ahead for a conventional painting. Many Dutch artists specialized in 'peep-shows' painted inside small boxes, which were viewed by putting one eye to a tiny hole in the box. These peep-shows created a very compelling trompe l'oeil.

The more bizarre examples of anamorphosis, like this one, were usually designed by graphical calculation of the distortion caused by the mirror, but some artists, particularly in China, worked empirically, simply painting while viewing the brush through the appropriate mirror. The distortion of anamorphosis was usually considered as little more than an amusing trick, but sometimes pictures like these were used to camouflage portraits that were forbidden for political reasons or to conceal pornographic pictures.

73

This eighteenth-century anonymous Dutch anamorphosis is seen correctly when viewed, from above, through a conical mirror placed in the centre, as seen on the right.

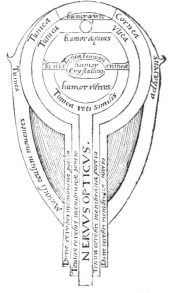

Alhazen's geometric diagram of the eye, c. 1000.

solid objects that they portray. The quest for perfection in the *trompe l'oeil* was one attempt to destroy the paradox of paintings.

It was the Romantic movement that suddenly rediscovered what pre-Renaissance iconographers must surely have known – that the picture itself is part of the perception it creates. Was abstraction in art an inevitable response to the discovery of paradox? Certainly it attempts to resolve the conflict by exploiting the painting as an object itself – almost the antithesis of the transparent reality of the *trompe l'oeil*. But to defy the model-builder in the mind, to try to express an idea independent of a subject, is even more difficult than mimicking reality. 'A good painter has two chief objects to paint', wrote Leonardo da Vinci, 'man and the intention of his soul; the former is easy, the latter hard.'

The fact that light forms an image on the retina posed serious problems for art; but the discovery of the retinal image presented difficulties no less profound for philosophy and science. The Arab, Ibn Al Haitham or Alhazen, described the convergence of rays of light on the eye in about 1000 A.D., and Christopher Scheiner carried out crude experiments on the optical properties

74

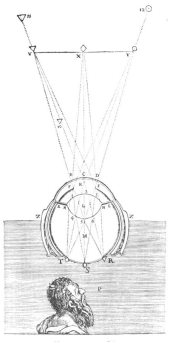

Descartes' illustration of his experimental observation of the image in an ox's eye, from La Dioptrique *of 1637, published in the same volume as* Discours de la Méthode, *in which he introduced the principle of Cartesian doubt.*

of the eye early in the seventeenth century. However, René Descartes usually takes the credit for the first accurate description of the retinal image. He took the eye of an ox, cut a window in the back of it and replaced it with paper. Holding the eye up to the light he saw on the paper a tiny inverted image of his room. I think it is no coincidence that he published this discovery in 1637, side by side with the first statement of his philosophical principle of believing nothing that he felt he might doubt. If the apparent richness of our visual world comes into us in such a comical form – a tiny picture, upside-down – how can we possibly trust it? The internalization of knowledge is a problem that has dogged philosophy, and physiology, ever since.

The British school of empiricist philosophy, from Francis Bacon and John Locke in the seventeenth century, to Bishop George Berkeley and David Hume in the eighteenth, did put their trust in sensory experience as a reliable source of knowledge. They saw around them the growing material success of England in trade and exploration. They recognized the power of scientists, like the brilliant experimenters Isaac Newton and Robert Boyle, to explain through observation. Observing events and gaining knowledge by inductive inference must be the only means by which we can discover truth.

But George Berkeley even became worried about the very existence of any material object outside the content of the mind. When we put our hands near a fire we feel pain; when we put sugar in our mouths we experience

Here Descartes shows how the retinal image (G, F, E), on the right, is an inverted picture of the true object.

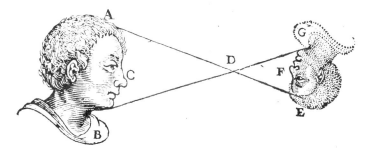

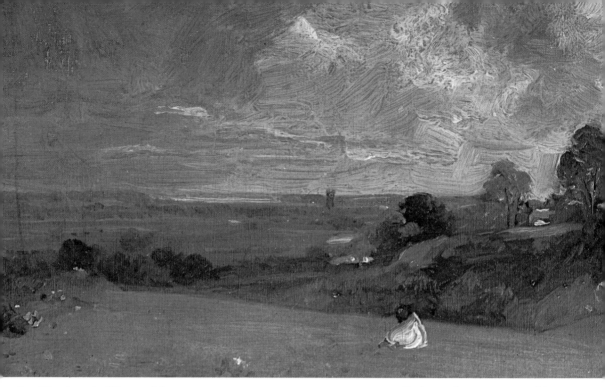

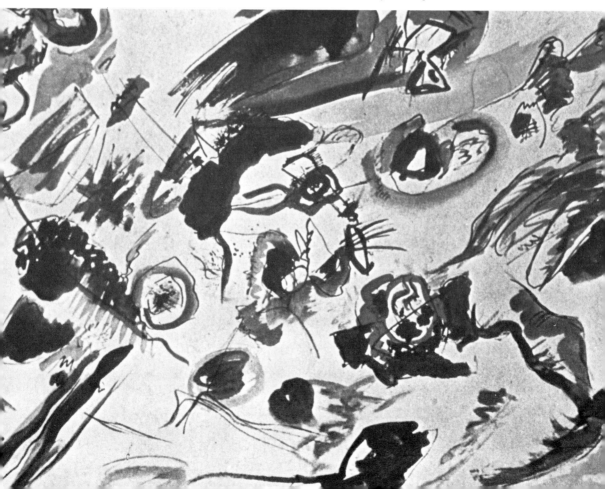

The picture itself is part of the perception it creates. 'Dedham from Langham', c. 1813, by John Constable.

Exploiting the painting as an object itself. 'First abstract', 1910, by Wassily Kandinsky.
© by SPADEM Paris, 1976.

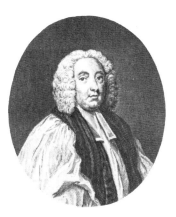

Bishop George Berkeley (1685–1753).

pleasure. But no-one could claim that fire contains pain or sugar pleasure. Then why should one think that any of our other sensations, of shape and colour, of loudness and tone, originate in the material properties of objects? By comparison with Descartes' dictum, '*cogito, ergo sum*', Berkeley retorted: '*esse est percipi*', to exist is to be perceived. But Bishop Berkeley did not conclude that objects disappeared when he turned his back on them, nor that his bedroom disintegrated when he blew his candle out. They must continue to exist because they are always observed by somebody else, someone who has to be everywhere at once. This theory of solipsism is admirably summarized in the famous limerick of Ronald Knox and its reply:

'There once was a man who said, "God
Must find it exceedingly odd
   If he finds that this tree
   Continues to be
When there's no one about in the quad."

Dear Sir, your astonishment's odd.
I am always about in the quad
   And that's why the tree
   Will continue to be
Since observed by,
       Yours faithfully, God.'

The problem of internal inference about the world, posed by Descartes, is certainly not solved even by modern brain research. Descartes himself avoided it neatly by imagining sensory nerves from the eyes, the ears and the skin terminating around the pineal gland in the brain, which he proposed as the principal home of the soul. Simply contacting the soul in this physical manner was enough; the soul was responsible for the actual seeing, hearing and feeling. Signals set up by the two eyes were even fused together to give a convenient *single*

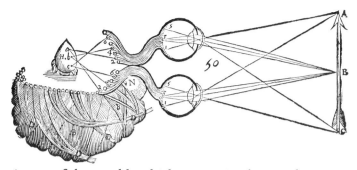

picture of the world, which was twisted around to turn the inverted retinal image the right way up again. But this is no solution, of course. It merely puts the task of recognition one step further on. There is no little man in the human brain to rush around looking at the signals from the senses. If there were, how would *his* eyes and ears work? Yet much of the physiological investigation of the brain has been concerned with the Cartesian problem of internal maps.

Like the cartographers of the Earth, who were so active at the time, neurologists and experimental physiologists in the second half of the last century were geographers of the mind. The British neurologist John Hughlings Jackson, working in London in the 1860s,

The localization of the main sensory and motor areas in the human brain. The labels have been added to a drawing of the left side of the brain made by the French anatomist, Louis Pierre Gratiolet (1815–1865), who named many of the convolutions of the cortex.
The motor cortex, occupying the pre-central gyrus in the frontal lobe, contains a map of the muscles of the opposite side of the body. Stimulation here causes jerky movements of these muscles. The somatic-sensory cortex, directly behind, in the post-central gyrus of the parietal lobe, has a similarly arranged map which receives sensory information from receptors in the skin, the joints, muscles and tendons. The auditory cortex, which plays a part in the analysis of sound, occupies the upper part of the temporal lobe. The primary visual cortex is mainly hidden from view on the inner surface of the back of the occipital lobe, but there are subsidiary visual areas that occupy the rest of the occipital lobe and probably spread down the sides of the temporal lobe.

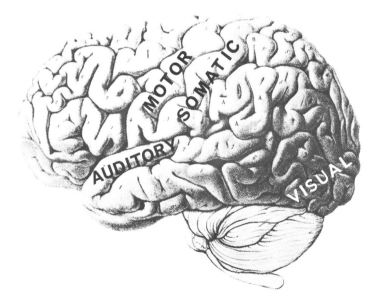

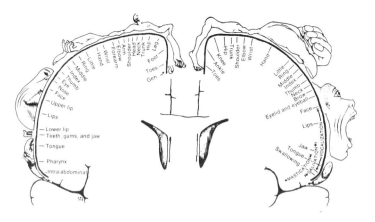

The motor homunculus, shown on the right, was first discovered by John Hughlings Jackson. Imagine the right side of the brain, sliced through the motor cortex. The cartoon of the body shows the order of representation of the muscles (opposite leg at the top of the motor strip, face at the bottom) and the relative amount of space devoted to each part (most for the fine muscles of the hands and lips).

The somatic-sensory homunculus, on the left, is arranged along the cortex directly behind the motor strip. It has much the same sequence of representation and exaggeration of certain features. These diagrams are modified from Figures 17 and 22 of Penfield and Rasmussen (1957).

discovered a new continent, in the brain. Some of his epileptic patients had fits that started with uncontrollable movements in one part of the body; the thumb of one hand, one of the toes or a corner of the mouth – and always in the same place. Now, epileptic convulsions are caused by irritation in the brain and Hughlings Jackson related the region of injury to the part of the body where the fits began. Thus he discovered what is now called the motor cortex – a strip of brain tissue on the side of the cerebral hemispheres, which represents the muscles on the opposite side of the body. The motor cortex is the keyboard of an instrument whose strings are the muscles, which finally play the melody of movement.

Other explorers soon made maps in different parts of the cortex for each of the senses. Directly behind the motor cortex is a second strip that receives a map of the entire body surface from the receptors in the skin. Again, it is as if the shape of the body were drawn out on the surface of the brain. And what did the physiologists call this body map? The *homunculus*! The little man! As if this picture of the body solved the paradox of Descartes!

But the cortical homunculus is a strangely inaccurate map. In it there is much more space devoted to man's face, his thumbs and his fingers than to his trunk and the

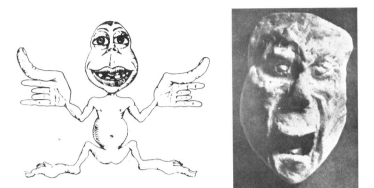

surface of his legs. When Edgar Adrian, now Lord
Adrian of Cambridge, recorded electrical activity from
the touch area in the pig's cortex, he found an even
odder map – a porcunculus, I suppose it should be
called. An enormous fraction of the pig's touch area is
dedicated to its snout. And in a mouse, the whiskers
occupy most of the touch cortex. The principle seems to
be that the most important and sensitive areas of the
body are most generously represented in the map.

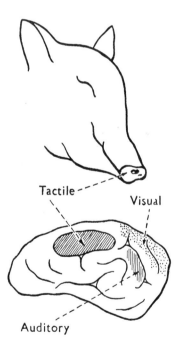

Tactile

Visual

Auditory

Adrian's drawing, in 1943, of the
huge area in the pig's somatic-
sensory cortex devoted to the
opposite half of its snout. This
patch alone is bigger than the entire
auditory cortex and as large as the
visual cortex.

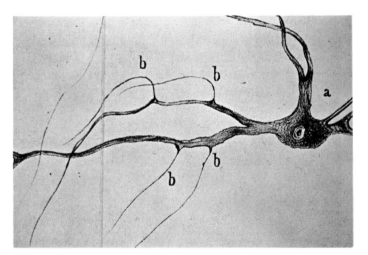

Otto Deiters, in 1865, drew the
first reasonably accurate diagrams
of the nerve cell body, its processes
(called dendrites) and its fibre or
axon. He painstakingly dissected
apart single nerve cells from the
spinal cord, probably of an ox, and
here he illustrates the axons (a),
together with other fine filaments (b)
apparently sprouting from the
dendrites. In fact the latter may
have been the termination of fibres
from other neurons ending on the
cell's dendrites.

80

This drawing, published by A. S. Dogiel in 1891, shows two nerve cells from the human retina. (The retina of the eye is structurally an outgrowth of the brain and it contains many interconnected nerve cells.) These are so-called ganglion cells whose fibres, or axons (a and a') leave the eye and pass into the optic nerve. Dogiel also shows the cells' dendrites (b), but draws them as if they literally connected together the protoplasm of the two cells without interruption. At the time there was a dominant idea amongst anatomists that the cells of the nervous system formed a continuous network or 'syncitium'.

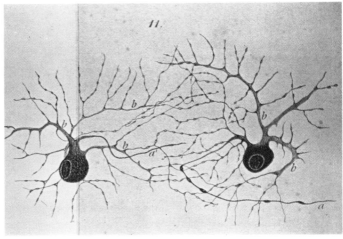

The nervous system is not a syncitium. The specialized junctions, called 'synapses', between the terminations of one axon and the dendrites or cell body of the next neuron, are minute but definite gaps, across which communication is usually mediated by a chemical transmitter. The substance is released by the terminals as impulses arrive and it diffuses across the synaptic gap to act on the membrane of the next cell. It either excites it, contributing to the setting off of an impulse, or inhibits it, reducing the chance of an impulse. The independence of nerve cells is demonstrated in this remarkable photo-micrograph by Akimichi Kaneko. It shows two so-called 'horizontal cells' in the retina of the dogfish eye. Kaneko succeeded in inserting fine glass recording electrodes into both tiny nerve cells at the same time and injected fluorescent dye from the electrodes to label the two cells. One is filled with yellow dye, the other with red. Their processes are clearly seen to be touching.

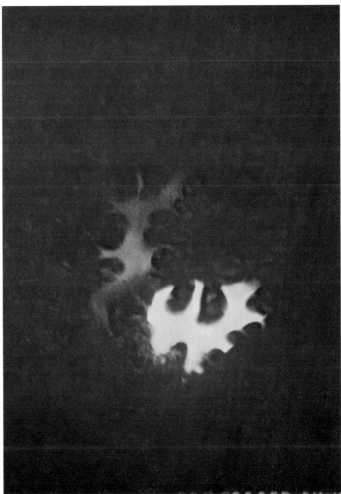

But not just the surface of the skin is sensed within the cortex. The very existence of the body is registered there as well. Injuries behind the touch area, in the *parietal lobe*, produce a most extraordinary disturbance of the relationship between body and mind. The opposite side of the body is simply lost to its owner's consciousness. It hangs as an unwanted parasite on his conceptual self. Patients with this condition shave only one side of their face, comb only half of their hair and they object to sharing their hospital bed with what they feel to be somebody else's arms and legs. The eminent Russian neurologist Alexander Luria transcribed the thoughts of a soldier Lev Zassetsky, who was injured in this part of his brain during the Second World War:

'Suddenly I'll come to, look to the right of me, and be horrified to discover half of my body is gone. I'm terrified; I try to figure out what's become of my right arm and leg, the entire right side of my body. I move the fingers of my left hand, feel them, but can't see the fingers of my right hand and somehow I'm not even aware they're there ... Often, I even forget where my forearm or buttocks are and have to think of what these two words refer to. I know what the word *shoulder* means and that the word *forearm* is closely related to it. But I always forget where my forearm is located. Is it near my neck or my hands? ...

'When the doctor says: "Hands on your hips!" I stand there wondering what this means. Or if he says: "Hands at your sides ... your sides ... hands at your sides ..." What does this mean?'

If we are to believe the Existentialist writer Jean-Paul Sartre, this personal sense of bodily existence can also be lost in the depths of terror. In his short story, 'The Wall', Sartre describes the sensations of a man awaiting execution during the Spanish Civil War:

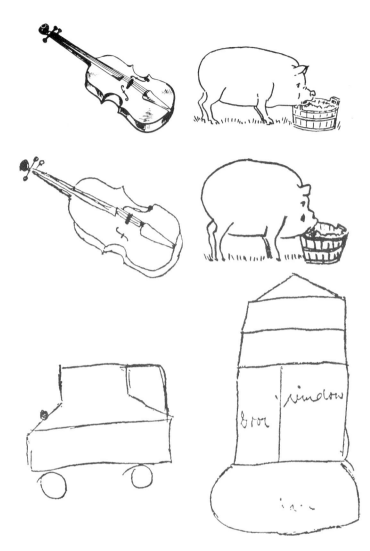

'My body, I saw with its eyes, I heard with its ears, but it was no longer me; it sweated and trembled by itself and I didn't recognize it any more. I had to touch it and look at it to find out what was happening, as if it were the body of someone else ... Everything that came from my body was all cockeyed. Most of the time it was quiet and I felt no more than a sort of weight, a filthy presence against me.'

Perhaps the most extraordinary map in the brain is the visual one, which Hermann Munk and Gordon

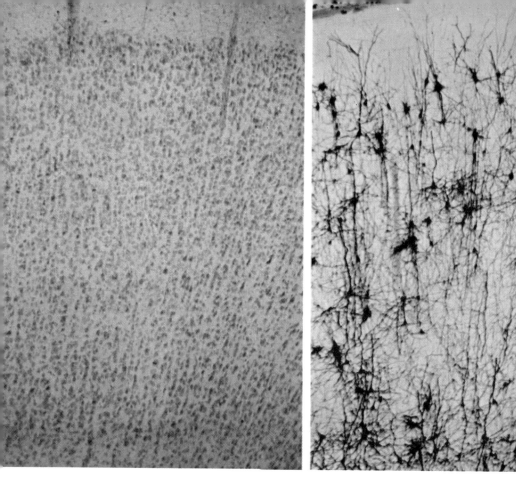

The astonishing tangle. These two photo-micrographs, made by Hendrik Van der Loos, are of successive microscopic sections, from the visual cortex of a rabbit. The surface of the cortex is towards the top and the entire depth of the cortex is about 2 mm. The first section, on the left, is stained with a dye that shows every nerve cell body as a blue dot. The second one is dyed by the Golgi method, which impregnates with black silver only about 2 per cent of all the cells but shows their dendrites and parts of their axons. Every cell on the left has connections as rich as those on the right!

Holmes first started to chart; in fact there is not just one map of the visual world but perhaps a dozen or more in a monkey, and presumably also in man. This amazing array of charts in the occipital and temporal lobes of the cortex is a veritable atlas of the world of vision. Each map has a different scale and like the various pages in a real atlas, showing geological structure, demographic data, rainfall and so on, the visual maps each emphasize a different component – colour in one, shape in another, movement in a third. Each time the eyes shift their gaze a new torrent of information pours through this labyrinth of maps.

Any injury to an individual portion of this visual atlas, beyond the primary area of Holmes and Munk, causes a partial loss of the description of the visual world – a kind of scotoma of knowledge. Damage in one place

84

might abolish colour perception alone; in another, the ability to see more than one thing at a time is lost; in another, whole objects cannot be recognized although all their individual parts are seen quite normally. And finally, brain damage can even steal the capacity to interpret a *real* map; the concepts of space are destroyed and the patient is lost even in his own home.

But just as a real map is not the country it portrays, so the sensory maps in the brain are not explanations for the objects of our perceptual world. For the source of knowledge, for the solution to Descartes' dilemma, we must look within the maps, at the nerve cells of which they are made – the neurons of knowledge. There are more than ten thousand million nerve cells in the human brain. Each cubic inch of the cerebral cortex probably contains more than ten thousand miles of nerve fibres, connecting the cells together. If the cells and fibres in one human brain were all stretched out end to end they would certainly reach to the moon and back. Yet the fact that they are *not* arranged end to end enabled man to go there himself. The astonishing *tangle* within our heads makes us what we are. Every cell in the cortex receives on its surface an average of several thousand terminals from the fibres of other cells. The richness of interconnection makes each neuron a Cartesian soul.

Lord Adrian made the first electrical recordings of the activity of individual nerve fibres, in Cambridge, in 1925. He discovered a universal law, one whose influence will, in the long run, be as important as Newton's laws of motion, for it would be impossible to understand the brain without this law: neurons communicate with each other by sending bursts of brief electrical pulses along their fibres. The pulses do not vary in size but only in the frequency of their bursts, which can be up to a thousand impulses in a second.

In the visual system, nerve cells look out at the world

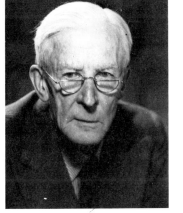

Lord Adrian of Cambridge.

through their connections from the one hundred million or more receptors in each eye. When physiologists turned their recording microelectrodes on these visual neurons, the results were a revelation. For each cell seemed not to be passively signalling the brightness or darkness of the retina, as we might expect, but to be searching for meaningful combinations of features, for the boundaries and shapes in the image that define the edges of objects.

One of the most remarkable of such experiments was reported in 1959 by the American Jerome Lettvin and his colleagues, in a scientific paper, which is already a classic, entitled 'What the frog's eye tells the frog's brain'. They recorded impulses from fibres in the frog's optic nerve and found that different classes of fibres would only respond with a burst of impulses if an appropriate pattern was projected on a screen in front of the eye. In other words, the eye has a language for its soliloquy to the brain. It speaks in symbols that define the important features of the visual scene. In the frog's optic nerve, to quote Lettvin, one class of fibre responds only 'to a small object passed through the field; the response does not outlast the passage; . . . the discharge is greater the greater the convexity . . . of the boundary of the dark object. . . . A smooth motion has less effect than a jerky one. . . . We have been tempted . . . to call [them] "bug perceivers".'

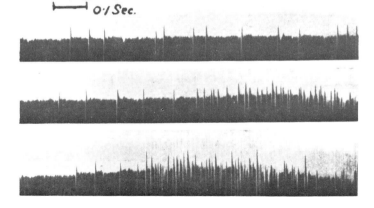

Some of Adrian's first recordings from very small numbers of individual nerve fibres. Each spiky deflection is a single nerve impulse. These records were taken from the sensory nerves of a cat's toe. The toe was flexed slowly, more quickly and very rapidly to produce these three traces. The frequency of firing depends on the strength of the stimulus – Adrian's law.

86

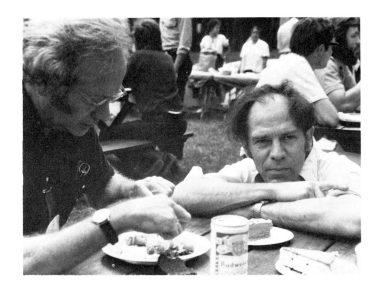

David Hubel (eating) and Torsten Wiesel (crouching), of Harvard Medical School, who described the 'feature-detecting' properties of nerve cells in the primary visual cortex of the cat and the monkey. They recorded impulses from individual cortical nerve cells in anaesthetized animals and projected simple patterns on a screen in front of the animals' eyes. Most of these cortical neurons are selectively sensitive to edges, moving with a particular orientation across a certain part of the visual field.

These experimental records of Hubel and Wiesel, photographed from an oscilloscope, show the impulses (vertical deflections) produced by a cell in the monkey's visual cortex. When no pattern was present on the screen this cell was totally silent (even if the overall illumination was turned on and off) but when a diagonal black line was moved to the right over a particular part of the screen the cell responded with a burst of impulses (see the first half of trace D). It gave only one impulse, however, when the same line moved back to the left (second half of trace D). If the angle of the moving line was changed by more than a few degrees (see other oscilloscope traces) the cell's response declined. Presumably cells like this are constantly chattering away in our brains, describing the appearance of the edges of objects in our visual fields, and hence helping us to recognize their shapes and patterns of movement.

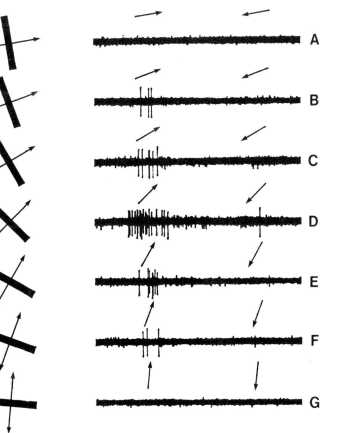

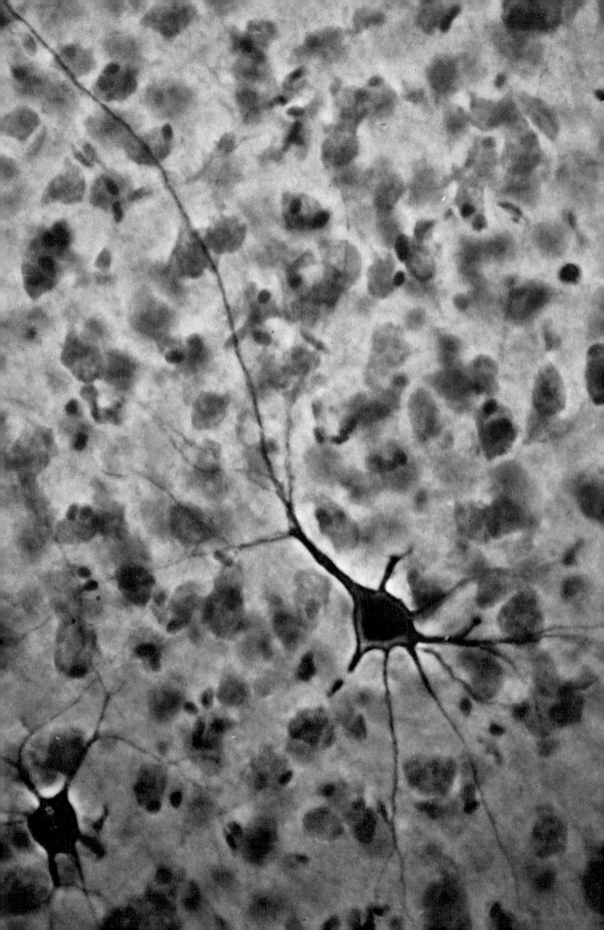

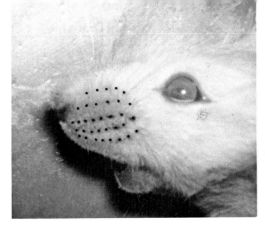

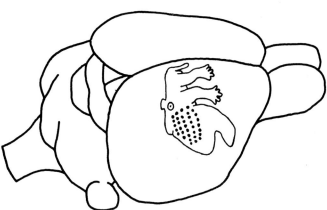

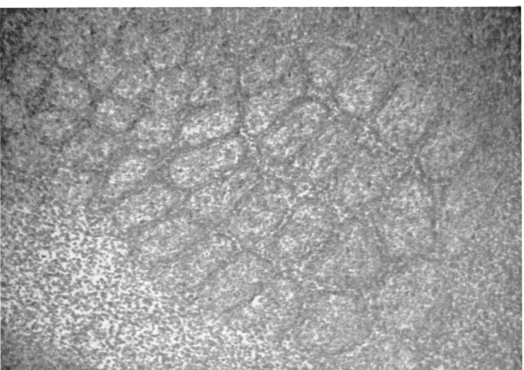

In the 'musculus' – the map of the body surface in the somatic-sensory cortex of a mouse – the representation of the whiskers on the muzzle occupies a very large fraction of the total body map. This is an example of the general rule that each cortical sensory region devotes a disproportionate area to the most acutely sensitive part of the sensory surface.

Cells in the visual cortex of the cat. The 'pyramidal' cell has a long dendrite that stretches towards the surfaces; the 'stellate' cell has a star-shaped pattern of dendrites. This micrograph was made by Giorgio Innocenti.

The photograph of the left side of the face of a mouse shows the pattern of insertion of the five rows of large whiskers. The musculus, drawn on the diagram of the right side of the brain, has an expanded representation for the head and particularly for the muzzle itself. Tom Woolsey and Hendrik Van der Loos discovered that, in the part of the cortex that represents the muzzle, the nerve cells of cortical layer 4 (where the incoming sensory fibres arrive) are organized in a remarkable way. The lower photograph is of a microscopic section of this area of the cortex, cut roughly parallel to the surface, through layer 4. The individual nerve cells appear as small blue-green dots and they are clearly grouped

together in rings, about 0·3 mm in diameter. These extraordinary collections of cells are called 'barrels', because their true three-dimensional appearance is like rows of barrels, filling layer 4. The 'walls' of each barrel consist of nerve cells that probably pick up signals from the mass of sensory fibres that arrives inside the barrel. The arrangement of barrels across the cortex matches exactly the pattern of whiskers in the mouse's moustache, so it is thought that each barrel might be the cortical representation of a single whisker. In fact, if one row of whiskers is removed in a new-born mouse, the appropriate row of barrels is missing in its cortex later in life.

No 'word' for a diagonal line. In the optic lobe of the octopus brain the anatomist J. Z. Young found that most of the dendrites of the cells that receive signals from the eye are spread in horizontal or vertical directions behind the eye, as shown in this micrograph from a thin section cut in the plane of the dendrites. These dendrites pick up incoming signals from the retinal image, and thus the cells presumably respond best to horizontal or vertical lines on the retina, not to diagonal. Indeed the psychologist Stuart Sutherland has shown that the octopus can learn to distinguish horizontal from vertical but cannot discriminate diagonal lines.

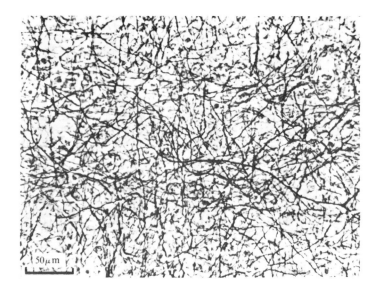

50μm

In the primary visual cortex of a monkey, neurons respond selectively to straight lines appearing in the visual field. Different cells signal different orientations of line. Each shape falling on the retina is described by the activity of these various line detectors. In the other visual areas of the cortex the combinations of activity from these line-detecting cells produce neurons that require the shape of a corner, or a particular type of movement or even the outline shape of a monkey's hand, appearing in the field, to make them spit out their spluttering messages to the rest of the brain.

The language of vision has a slightly different dialect for every species. The octopus probably has no 'word' for a diagonal line: it can only detect horizontal and vertical ones. Many animals have little or no ability to discriminate colour. But equally, some other species have nerve cells that can describe events that are invisible to us. A rabbit can see movement as slow as that of the sun across the sky. Some animals can detect the plane of polarisation of light or the direction of a magnetic field. We deceive ourselves if we think that our perceptual world is complete. It is what our neurons are able to tell us.

90

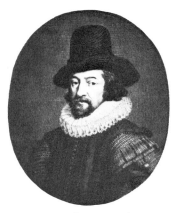

Francis Bacon (1561–1626).

We seem driven to say that such neurons have knowledge. They have intelligence, for they are able to estimate the probability of outside events – events that are important to the animal in question. And the brain gains its knowledge by a process analogous to the inductive reasoning of the classical scientific method. Neurons present arguments to the brain based on the specific features that they detect, arguments on which the brain constructs its hypothesis of perception. It was Francis Bacon, founder of the philosophical school of empiricism, who first recommended clearly the inductive method for the formulation of scientific theories. The classical method of science was surely inspired by the example of human perception!

Indeed, science itself can be regarded as a cultural extension of the biological process of acquiring knowledge. But even perception cannot proceed without *expectations*, built into the brain in the form of the experiences with which it is familiar. Equally, science has not progressed by induction alone. The '*anticipatio mentis*', the prejudice of insight, which Francis Bacon so much detested, is an essential part of science, just as it is of human perception.

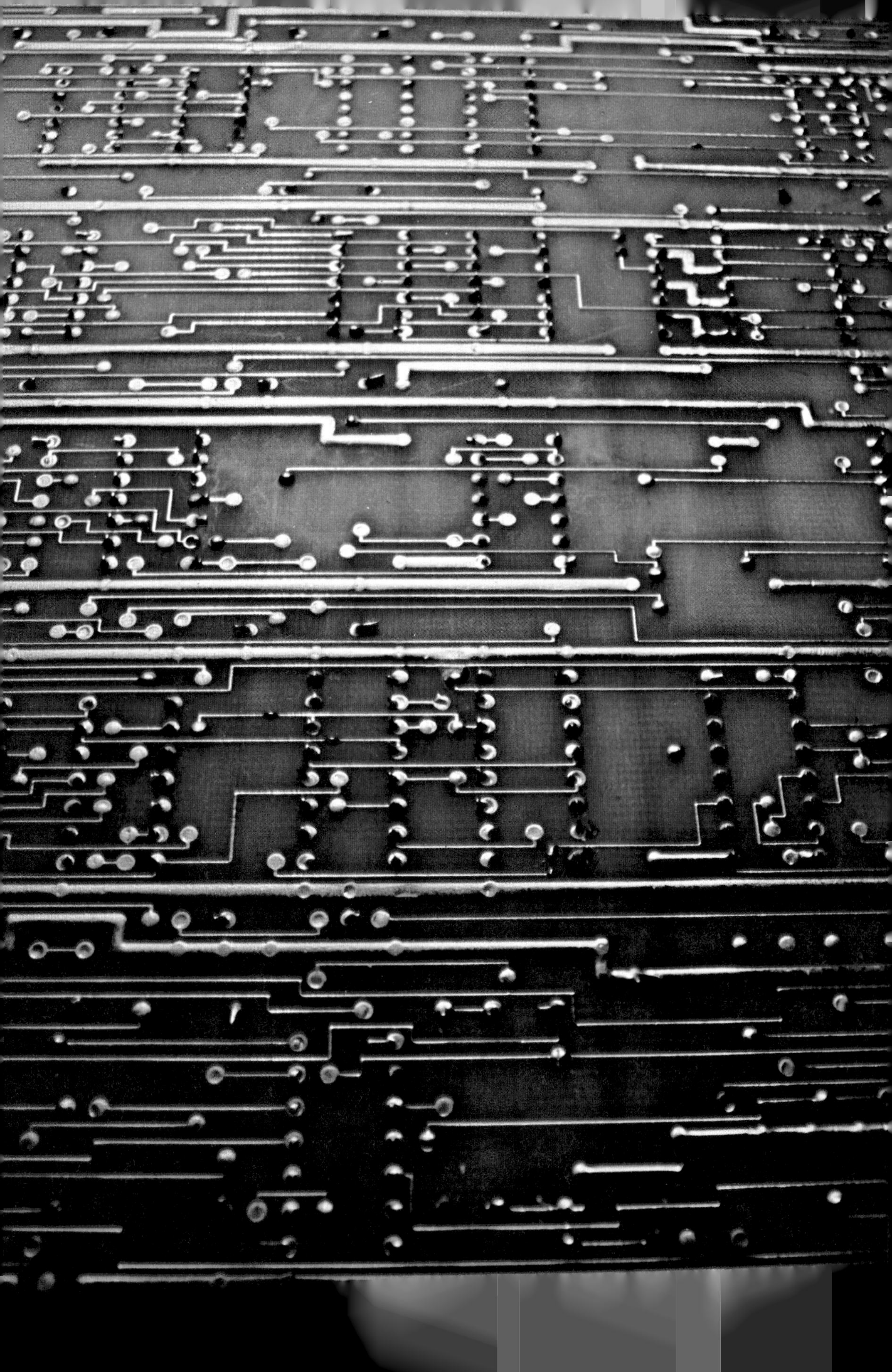

4 A child of the moment

> *'Remember thee?*
> *Ay thou poor ghost whiles memory holds a seat*
> *In this distracted globe. Remember thee?*
> *Yea, from the table of my memory*
> *I'll wipe away all trivial fond records,*
> *All saws of books, all forms, all pressures past*
> *That youth and observation copied there,*
> *And thy commandment all alone shall live*
> *Within the book and volume of my brain*
> *Unmixed with baser matter – yes by heaven!'*
> William Shakespeare, *Hamlet* (1.5)

Imagine that you are asked to remember the number '584'. What could be easier? Whether you wanted to or not, the number would be yours to recall for the next few minutes. With the slightest effort of will you could remember it at the end of this chapter; and, if it were important enough, you would recollect it next month, next year or next century.

There is an American – let us call him Henry M. – who has been robbed of this precious power to remember; not partially and gradually, just by growing old, as most of us will be; but suddenly and almost totally, by the knife of a well-intentioned surgeon. From Henry we can learn about the nightmare of eternal forgetfulness – a condition that Franz Kafka would have been delighted to describe. Brenda Milner, at the Montreal Neurological Institute, has followed the case of Henry for more than 20 years. She once asked *him* to try to remember

Memory circuit boards in a Honeywell Series 60 Level 6 minicomputer. They have capacity for 65,536 words of memory, yet are contained in a unit only 5¼ inches high and 15 inches wide. Solid-state memory units are gradually replacing ferrite-ring core memory in computer design.

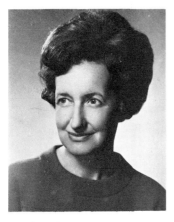

Brenda Milner.

that very number, '584'. He sat quietly, entirely un-distracted, for 15 minutes, and, to her surprise he, *could* recall the number. But when asked how he did it, this is what he said:

'It's easy. You just remember 8. You see, 5, 8 and 4 add up to 17. You remember 8; subtract it from 17 and it leaves 9. Divide 9 in half and you get 5 and 4, and there you are: 584. Easy!'

Henry lives in a world of his own, restricted not just in space but in time. Ever since an operation on his brain in 1953, his world has been just a few minutes long. Without such elaborate and fantastic tricks of rehearsal, almost everything slips from his mind, like water through a sieve. Every moment has a terrible freshness. He never knows the day of the week, what year it is or even his own age. Even though Brenda Milner has spent count-less hours with Henry, she is an utter stranger to him, and on each new occasion that they meet it is as if she were entering his transient world for the first time.

Henry works in a state rehabilitation centre, mount-ing cigarette lighters on cardboard frames, a task that he has learned to do skilfully. But still he can give no account whatever of his place of work how he gets there or the type of job that he does. So Henry has not lost the ability to learn new skills of *movement*; he is, quite simply, unable to remember the new contents of his *conscious* experience. His general intelligence is not at all reduced and he is painfully aware of his own short-

Examples from a memory test devised by Gollin (1960). The experimenter shows a patient a series of drawings, each one containing more detail than the last. The patient's task is to recognize the object from the earliest possible picture in the series. Hours or days later a normal person, when shown the same sets of cards, will identify the object at a much earlier stage in each series. Henry M. also shows some evidence of long-term remembering on this task, although he has no conscious recollection of having taken the test before. His deficiency may be one of consciously recalling stored information, not in laying down the store.

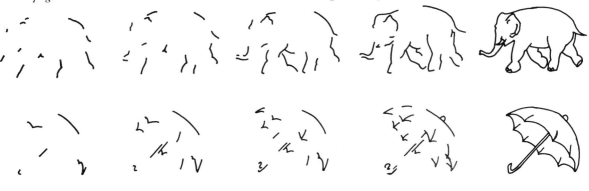

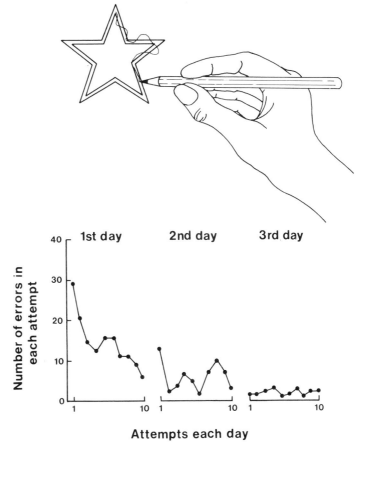

Henry M. shows definite improvement in any task involving learning skilled movements. In this test he was taught to trace between the two outlines of the shape of a star, while viewing his hand in a mirror. He improved considerably with each fresh test, although once again he had no idea that he had ever done the task before. (The graph plots the number of times, in each trial, that he strayed outside the outlines as he drew the star.)

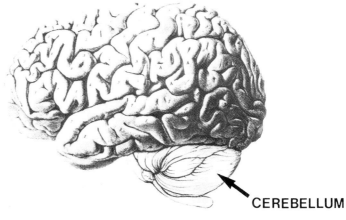

'Motor memory' for learning skilled movement may occur in the cerebellum, indicated on the drawing of the brain. Conscious perceptual and verbal memories, however, presumably involve the cerebral hemispheres and especially the hippocampus.

CEREBELLUM

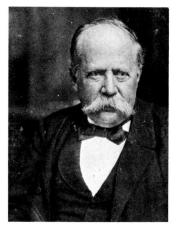

Friedrich Goltz (1834–1902).

comings. He apologizes constantly for the absence of his mind. 'Right now, I'm wondering', he once said, 'have I done or said anything amiss? You see, at this moment everything looks clear to me, but what happened just before? That's what worries me. It's like waking from a dream; I just don't remember.' . . . 'Every day is alone in itself, whatever enjoyment I've had, and whatever sorrow I've had.'

Henry still has his very old memories and habits, but cannot form new ones and even had amnesia for things that happened in the years immediately before the operation. Three years before, his favourite uncle died, but Henry suffers the same grief anew each time he is told of his uncle's death.

In 1892 the German physiologist Friedrich Goltz described a similar loss of memory in dogs after the cerebral cortex had been damaged. 'They do not learn from past experience', Goltz wrote. 'They do not *have* experiences, for only he who has memories can have experiences. The decerebrated dog is essentially nothing but a child of the moment.' Henry is a 'child of the moment', too; he is trapped, interminably, in the naïveté of infancy.

We discover from this special case that our memories have two forms: one of them is quickly created but fades within a few minutes, to be followed by a more persistent store, which can last for a lifetime. The most popular view is that short-term memories are converted or consolidated into the long-term ones, but it is just as possible that the two processes are totally independent. One thing seems certain; the embodiments of the two sorts of memory must be quite different. Henry has lost the power to form new long-term memories; or perhaps he *can* make them, but has no way to retrieve them again.

The injury to the brain of Henry was deliberate. When he was young he gradually developed epilepsy so severe that he was unable to work. The surgeon treating

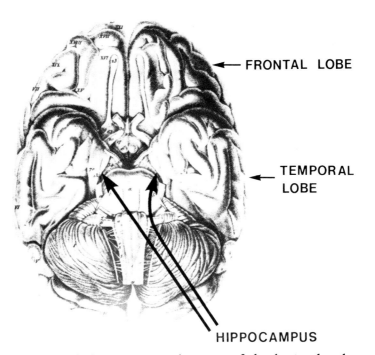

FRONTAL LOBE

TEMPORAL LOBE

HIPPOCAMPUS

The hippocampus is out of sight, folded under the inner surface of the temporal lobes, which are seen here in a drawing of the underside of the human brain by the phrenologist, Franz Joseph Gall.

him decided to remove the part of the brain that he thought was causing the epileptic seizures – an evolutionary ancient part of the cerebral cortex, called the hippocampus (meaning a seahorse, because of its twisted shape), which lies tucked inside the temporal lobes of the cerebral hemispheres. The hippocampus had been removed on one side in many previous patients, but because Henry's epileptic attacks seemed to involve the whole of his brain, the surgeon destroyed the hippocampus on both sides. And that was the cause of his present terrible state, for the hippocampus of man is crucially important in laying down or retrieving long-term memories. Presumably this surgical procedure will never be used again. Experimental brain surgery is perhaps the riskiest form of experimental medicine, because it is irreversible and its effects are expressed as changes in the personal experience and the behaviour of the patients involved. But it is also the area of medical practice that is least regulated by legislative control.

In the 1940s, as the epilepsy of Henry was becoming

97

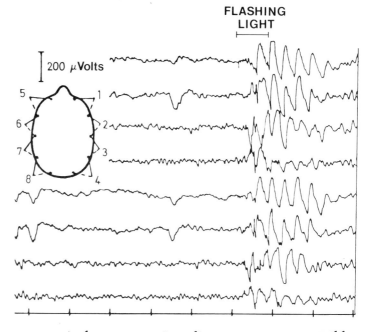

200 μVolts

An EEG recording from a seven-year-old boy reveals the storm of electrical waves that heralds the start of an epileptic seizure. The EEG was recorded separately from eight pairs of electrodes, seen in the drawing of the top of the head; the eight EEG traces show these simultaneous recordings. The deflections on the bottom trace occur once a second. The top trace indicates a burst of flashing lights that was shone into the boy's eyes for about one second. It triggers off rhythmic, low-frequency waves in the EEG, typical of an epileptic discharge. This boy suffered occasional fits while watching television, because of the flicker of the screen.

progressively worse, a Canadian neurosurgeon, Wilder Penfield, was gathering other evidence that the temporal lobes of man conceal the key to his memory. Penfield was also operating on epileptic patients, removing the areas of irritative damage in their brains. To guide him in pinpointing the epileptic focus he used a method of exploring the human brain that has provided perhaps more evidence about its organization than any other technique. He stimulated the surface of the brain with a weak electric current, not to damage it, but to excite impulses in the cells and fibres under the stimulating electrode. His patients were completely conscious during this electrical invasion of their minds. Only the scalp was locally anaesthetized; the tissue of the brain itself is insensible to touch, heat or pain.

Penfield hoped to discover in each patient an area in the brain which, upon stimulation, would arouse the same curious mental aura that ushered in the epileptic attacks. That would be the spot to destroy, Penfield argued; and this approach was remarkably successful. But it also gave him the chance to discover the functions

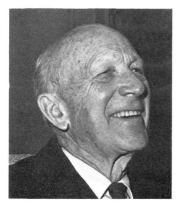

Wilder Penfield (1891–1976).

of other parts of the cerebral cortex. Stimulation of the motor cortex caused jerky twitches of the muscles, which the patient could not control; excitation of the touch area produced strange sensations felt by the patient in his skin; stimulation of the visual cortex made the patient see flashes of light or swirling coloured forms in his visual field. But when Penfield moved his stimulating electrode to the temporal lobe and the hippocampus itself, the experiences of the patient were not mere fragments of movement or sensation. They were whole episodes of existence, plucked from the patient's previous life. The person would suddenly be transported into the past and would feel himself eavesdropping on a familiar scene.

One of Penfield's patients was a young woman. As the stimulating electrode touched a spot on her temporal lobe she cried out, 'I think I heard a mother calling her little boy somewhere. It seemed to be something that happened years ago . . . in the neighbourhood where I live.' A moment later the same spot was stimulated. 'Yes', she said, 'I hear the same familiar sounds; it seems to be a woman calling; the same lady.' Then the elec-

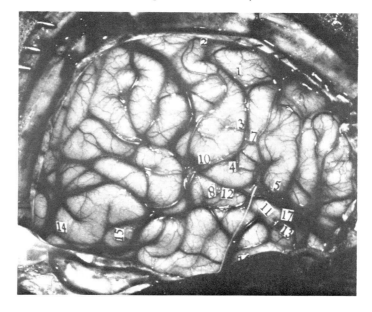

During one of Penfield's operations, described in the text, the right temporal lobe of a young woman was exposed and electrically stimulated at the places marked with numbered tags. The woman was fully conscious and described her curious sensations. The recollection of a mother calling her child was evoked by stimulation at the spot marked 11 and that of a circus from the spot marked 13.

99

Several research groups around the world are trying to develop a prosthesis for the blind, utilizing the sensations produced by direct electrical stimulation of the visual cortex. G. S. Brindley and W. Lewin in London were the first to implant an array of stimulating electrodes over the brain of a blind patient. The X-ray picture shows an implant made by William Dobelle and his colleagues in Salt Lake City. A cable of wires running under the skin of the scalp connects the battery of electrodes to a socket bolted to the skull. A plug inserted into this socket transmits signals from a computer to stimulate the electrodes, which lie in an 8 by 8 matrix over the brain. As each one is stimulated the blind patient perceives a bright flash, a 'phosphene', which seems to him to be localized in a particular place in his blind visual field. The eye is by-passed, but the brain had no way of knowing that the signal is not coming from a real object in space. Different electrodes produce phosphenes at different points in the visual field. Dobelle and his team have chosen six of the electrodes, which produce a distribution of six phosphenes in a rectangle in the field, like the points of the 'Braille cell' – the pattern of dots used to represent letters in the Braille alphabet. By stimulating the correct combinations of electrodes they can transmit Braille letters to the patient who can read them rather faster than he can read with his finger tips. However, the long-term prospects for this technique seem very restricted. It is clearly extremely costly, even somewhat dangerous, and may be appropriate for only a small number of patients.

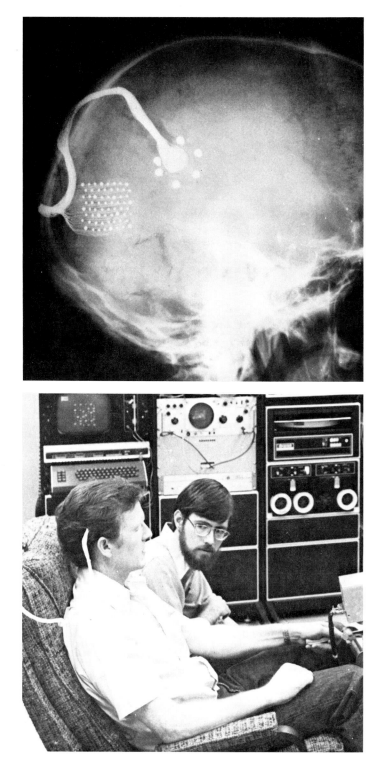

100

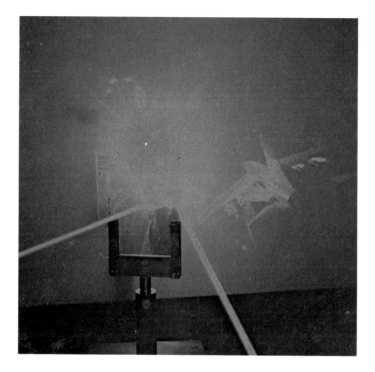

A three-dimensional image of an aeroplane is reproduced by shining light from a laser through a holographic plate. The plate itself, called a hologram, is made by illuminating a real, solid object with a bright beam of coherent laser light. The reflected light strikes the photographic plate, where it forms a complex interference pattern by mixing with a second beam of laser light shining directly on to the plate. The interference pattern, recorded on the developed hologram, contains information about the object; when it is illuminated once again by the direct beam of laser light the emerging rays recreate exactly the pattern of light that emanated from the original object. The solid object is seen just as if it were really present.

Because the information from each part of the object contributes to the interference pattern across the whole plate, the stored information is said to be 'distributed'. If part of the plate is broken off, the remaining portion still contains some information about the entire scene, degraded in quality in proportion to the amount of the plate that is missing.

trode was moved a little and she said, 'I hear voices. It is late at night, around the carnival somewhere – some sort of travelling circus. I just saw lots of big wagons that they use to haul animals in.'

There can be little doubt that Wilder Penfield's electrodes were arousing activity in the hippocampus, within the temporal lobe, jerking out distant and intimate memories from the patient's stream of consciousness.

Memory, its physical structure, is an unsolved challenge. It is, perhaps, the *central* question, rather like the problem of the structure of DNA, deoxyribonucleic acid, for molecular biology and genetics. But theories about the nature of memory have still not really progressed beyond the stage of description through analogy. Analogy has often been a valuable step in the discussion of biological problems, but it is, of its nature, constrained by the technological development of the time or the level of scientific knowledge in other fields. The restrictive nature of argument by analogy is aptly illus-

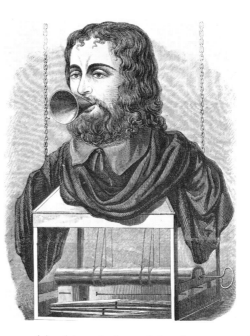

trated by historical models of memory. They are almost
all based on the devices used by man himself to store
information.

According to Aristotle, sensory impressions entered
the head with such force that they left physical inscrip-
tions in the brain, like a scribe engraving on a wax
tablet. This idea, that the mind is a *tabula rasa* on which
experiences are literally written, was espoused by the
Empiricist school of philosophy. 'Let us then suppose
the mind to be, as we say, white paper, void of all
characters, without any ideas'; wrote John Locke in
1690, 'how comes it to be furnished? Whence comes it
by that vast store, which the busy and boundless fancy
of man has painted on it with an almost endless variety?
... To this I answer in one word, from experience.'

Even current models of memory dwell on analogies
with existing, artificial methods of storing information.
Mental memory has been compared with the electro-
magnetic polarization of ferrite rings in the core memory
of a computer, and with the 'distributed' image of a
hologram – a device that stores a record of a three-

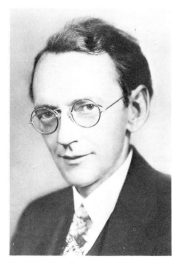
Karl Lashley (1890–1958).

dimensional scene by photographing the interference pattern produced by illuminating it with laser light.

Each analogy has a certain attraction because it mirrors some particular special feature of memory. The permanence of lines scratched in a wax tablet or written on paper mimicks the durability of real memory. The speed of access to the memory of a computer core is reminiscent of the remarkably rapid way in which neuronal memory can be consulted.

Because the information in a holographic plate is 'distributed', a somewhat degraded reconstruction of the entire stored image can still be retrieved even when part of the plate is destroyed. Now the psychologist Karl Lashley, working in the first half of this century, described a similar kind of resistance to local injury in the store of information in the rat's brain. The actual representation of remembered events is almost certainly in the cerebral cortex, but Lashley found that small areas of damage in the rat's cortex simply blurred the animal's ability to perform tasks that it had previously learned. The degree of degradation of memory was roughly proportional to the area of damaged cortex. He concluded that the cerebral hemispheres have a kind of 'mass action' in the remembering process. In the same way, the steady attrition of about 50,000 nerve cells that unavoidably die each day in the cerebral cortex of man does not rob us, piecemeal, of individual elements of memory; it gradually removes the edge from remembered events and stunts the power to capture new ones. Lashley expressed his frustration in failing to track down the physical substance of individual stored remembrances in a famous scientific paper in 1950. 'I sometimes feel,' he wrote, 'in reviewing the evidence on the localization of the memory trace, that the necessary conclusion is that learning just is not possible.'

Description by analogy seems less successful for the nervous system than for other organs in the body. The

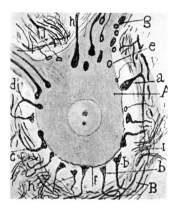

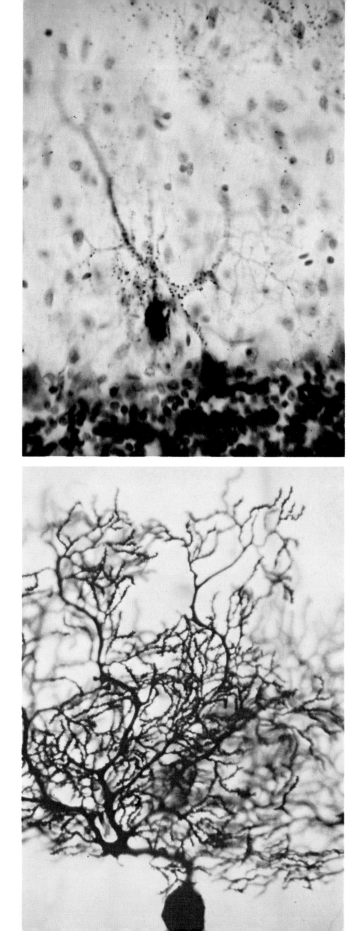

The change in physical structure
that embodies long-term memory
may take place at the terminals of
axons ending on the dendrites or cell
body of the next cell in the chain.
This diagram, by the Great Spanish
neuro-anatomist Santiago Ramón y
Cajal (1852–1934), shows the
terminals ending on a nerve cell
body. Cajal worked to disprove the
idea that the brain is a syncitium
of cells in protoplasmic continuity;
he believed that synaptic junctions
were extremely important in the
regulation of nervous transmission.
Changes in the efficiency of
synapses might underlie the
storage of information in the brain.

A Purkinje cell from the rabbit's
cerebellum appears in all its glory
in this photomicrograph made by
Hendrik van der Loos. The cell has
been stained with silver by the Golgi
method, which reveals the full
extent of its 'tree' of dendrites.
Many nerve fibres terminate on tiny
twigs, called 'dendritic spines',
which can be seen all over the
dendrites. The axon of the Purkinje
cell emerges from the bottom right of
the cell body.

The terminals on a real nerve cell are revealed by a modern technique. This micrograph, prepared by Michael Murphy and James O'Leary, shows the yellow-coloured dendrites of two large 'Purkinje cells' in the cerebellum of a cat. The smaller blue-black shapes at the bottom of the picture are other types of nerve cells. A radio-actively labelled amino acid has been injected elsewhere in the brain, amongst cells whose fibres terminate on Purkinje cells. The radioactivity has travelled along the axons and collected in the terminals. A photographic process reveals the radioactivity as black dots, marking the terminals, scattered over the dendrites of the Purkinje cells. Changes in the efficiency of certain synaptic contacts on the cells of the cerebellum may be involved in motor learning.

A micrograph taken with an electron microscope of a tiny area in the visual cortex of a cat. The dendrite of a stellate cell runs across the picture and four synaptic terminals are seen ending on the right-hand side of this dendrite. The upper three terminals (E), each less than 1/1000 mm in diameter, are probably excitatory ones; they are recognized by their small round vesicles, containing transmitter substance, and the thickening of the membranes around the synaptic gap (shown by arrows). A nerve fibre, or axon, that probably leads to the uppermost terminal is also visible. The lowest terminal (I) has somewhat flattened vesicles within it and a slightly different membrane thickening; it may be an inhibitory terminal, whose transmitter substance would tend to oppose the excitatory influence of the transmitter substance from the neighbouring excitatory terminals. Electron-micrograph by Laurence Garey.

heart is *like* a pump in its action and the kidney is *like* a filter because they *are* a pump and a filter. The analogies are both comparisons with other pieces of machinery and actual explicit descriptions of the mechanism of heart and kidney. But however similar in its properties mental memory is to a computer core or a hologram, the brain is *not* a set of magnetized rings or a laser-illuminated photographic plate. The value of analogy is that it provides rules, best expressed in mathematical terms, for accomplishing certain logical processes. The rules will restrict the set of possible devices that can accomplish the task. Unfortunately, the physical structure and mechanisms of operation in the brain are so unlike those of any piece of machinery made by man that analogies are usually weak.

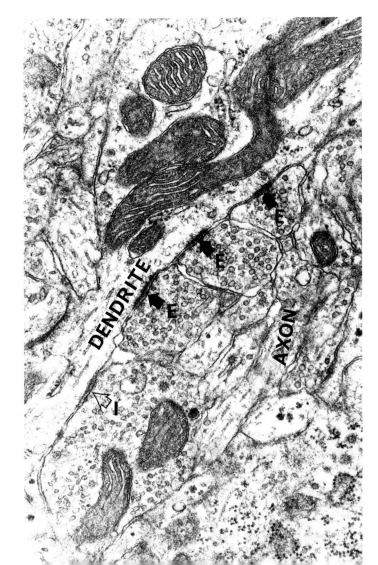

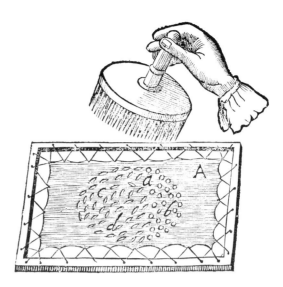

René Descartes's analogy for mental memory (from the Traité de l'Homme, 1664) was characteristically original and remarkably far-sighted. He imagined that the passage of vital spirit through certain pores in the ventricle wall would force open those pores and produce a persistent representation of the original pattern of activity; this was the form of mental memory, he proposed. In this diagram he compares the process to the impression of a pattern of holes made in a linen cloth by punching it with a set of needles. When the needles are withdrawn, the holes stay completely or partially open. He also tried to explain the fact that recall of a particular remembrance is assisted by partial information about it: Descartes said that if just some of the holes in the linen were to be re-opened 'that fact alone could cause others . . . to re-open at the very same time, especially if they had all been opened several times together . . . For example, if I see two eyes with a nose, I at once imagine a forehead, and a mouth and all the other parts of a face.'

In any case, most theories of memory, whether couched in terms of mere analogy, or even in terms of the storage of information in networks of real nerve cells, concentrate on the manner in which events can cause changes in physical structures. In other words, they are concerned with the *machinery* of memory, not the *code* – the symbolic form in which the events are registered. The printing of words on a page is a simple and efficient method of storing information, but it means nothing without knowledge of the language in which the message is written. Most theories of memory are, as it were, concerned with the question of ink and paper and not with the much more fundamental issue of the grammar of remembrance.

From this point of view, the most compelling theory of memory is the claim that remembering might consist of the synthesis of specific chemical molecules in the brain, the structure of each molecule representing a remembered event. This hypothesis is so powerful because it not only describes a possible physical substrate for memory (the synthesized molecule), but also embodies the nature of the code by which the information might be stored (the sequence of compounds in the molecule or its specific shape).

Certainly, long-term memory must involve some physical change in the structure of the brain. Consider the following classical experiment: a rat is quickly taught to run a maze or perform some other task. It is then cooled down to about 5°C for some time, stopping all electrical activity in its brain. When it thaws out, the rat, none the worse for wear, tries the maze again. With a fairly long interval between learning and cooling, the rat still remembers the maze. But if cooled within minutes or perhaps seconds of learning, it reacts as if the task were completely new. The necessary conclusion is that the initial storage of information, short-term memory, involves on-going patterns of nerve impulses in circuits of nerve cells connected together by their fibres, while long-term memory is a lasting structural change in the pathway of cells. Some would say that this structural change is the synthesis of a substance that actually describes the remembered event. The theory of chemical memory even contains a strong analogy, for it draws a comparison between mental memory and that other monolithic biological mechanism of remembering – the genetic code.

The double helix of DNA, the genetic code, is indeed a store of information. What it remembers is the exact chemical composition of the organic species it belongs to; it is, quite simply, a recipe for replicating the structure of that organism. And the sequence of nucleotide bases within the double helix is not just the *structure* of genetic memory but is the *code* as well. The four different bases that constitute the nucleotide chain are letters in an alphabet. Each triplet of three successive bases forms a word that specifies a particular amino acid. The amino acids, of which there are twenty kinds, are assembled according to the instructions written in each gene, to make a polypeptide chain, which folds

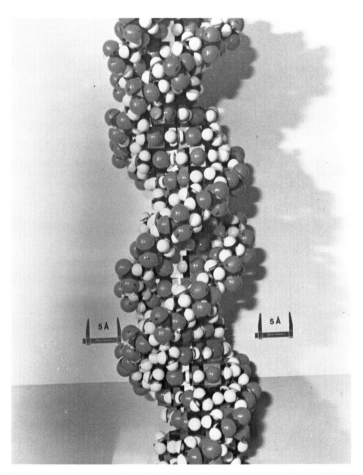

A model of a small part of the DNA molecule. Nucleotide bases arranged in pairs form the centre of the spiral, with a helix of sugars running around them. The string of bases specifies sequences of amino acids for the construction of protein molecules.

into a protein molecule. It is these proteins that define the nature and form of each organism; in particular, the enzyme proteins determine the metabolic processes that the cell can perform.

The structure of DNA proposed by Francis Crick and James Watson has put flesh on the skeleton that Charles Darwin left in the Victorians' cupboard. It explains, with such staggering simplicity, the physical nature of genetic memory, *and* the code by which it stores information. What Darwin had supplied, a hundred years before, was the other essential component – a way in which genetic memories could be *forgotten*. Natural selection is the mechanism by which only useful genetic memories are retained.

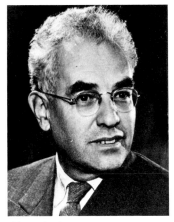

Alexander Luria.

It is difficult to exaggerate the importance of *forgetting* in *mental* memory, too. The selection process that lets us store in long-term memory only a tiny fraction of the running contents of short-term memory is essential if the brain is to use particular instances to derive general principles, by a process of inference. The Russian psychologist Alexander Luria has described a man whose memory seemed to have no limit – a mnemonist whose mind was so extraordinary that Luria wrote of him in terms reserved for the mentally ill. He could commit to memory in a couple of minutes a table of fifty numbers, which he could recall in every minute detail many years later. His greatest difficulty was in learning how to forget the endless trivia that cluttered his mind.

In a remarkable short story, *Funes the Memorious*, the

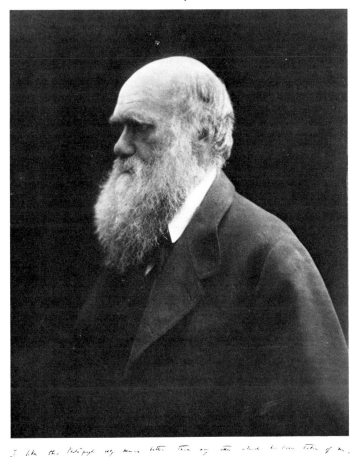

Charles Darwin (1809–1882). A copy of this photograph, below which Darwin wrote 'I like this photograph very much better than any other which has been taken of me', was presented to Chairman Mao Tse-tung by Edward Heath.

Argentinian writer Jorge Borges describes, in fiction, the alien totality of forgetlessness. A young boy, Ireneo Funes, had a fall from a horse and forgot how to forget. Borges writes:

'On falling from the horse, he lost consciousness; when he recovered it, the present was almost intolerable, it was so rich and bright; the same was true of the most ancient and most trivial memories . . . We, in a glance, perceive three wine glasses on the table: Funes saw all the shoots, clusters, and grapes of the vine. He remembered the shapes of the clouds in the south at dawn on the 30th of April of 1882, and he could compare them in his recollection with the marbled grain in the design of a leather-bound book which he had seen only once, and with the lines in the spray which an oar raised in the Rio Negro on the eve of the battle of Quebracho . . . He told me: I have more memories in myself alone than all men have had since the world was a world.'

If remembering does include the laying down of molecular descriptions, the single most important part of the process, the selection of which events are worthy of long-term storage, must be done before they are committed to molecular memory.

But what kind of molecules in the brain could possibly qualify as the repository of mental memory? They would need to be complex and therefore large in order to have sufficient variability in form to represent the high informational content of each remembrance. Then the choice of appropriate macromolecules within the nerve cell is rather limited. They would have to be either proteins or the nucleic acids themselves – that is DNA, or RNA, the ribonucleic acid that transcribes the message from the DNA of the gene and which actually assembles the protein molecules. But all of these substances, DNA, RNA and protein, employ logically equivalent coded messages. The series of amino acids in a protein contains identical information to the sequence of bases in the RNA on which it grew, and this in turn is simply a re-coded version of the base sequence in the DNA of the gene. It is rather like the same sentence being expressed first in written words, then in Braille translation, and finally in Morse code; the information is identical. And so it is in protein, RNA and DNA.

In order for a wholly novel and unique protein or RNA molecule to be made for each memory, a new DNA sequence would have to be synthesized first, within the actual gene. But there is no evidence that the DNA of nerve cells is continuously changing. In fact DNA is virtually the only material that is *not* constantly being replaced in the living cell. The very permanence of genetic memory relies on the extraordinary stability of the DNA molecule; how can mental memory work by changing it?

There seem to be only two possible solutions to this dilemma. Either the whole theory of chemical memory is wrong, or the *existing*, inherited DNA of the genes already contains the capacity to synthesize the RNA or protein that is used to represent *any* conceivable new remembrance. Each brain might contain within itself all the potential memories that it could ever form; every event would merely trigger production of the appropriate molecule, which was already described, in latent form, in the animal's inherited DNA. In these terms, the evolution of the capacity to remember and to learn, and hence of intelligence itself, would consist of the generation, by mutation, of new DNA sequences that would represent hitherto undreamed-of memories.

This fantastic notion that every memory is innately within us, in our genetic make-up, is curiously reminiscent of Plato's nativist theory that all human knowledge is derived by the soul from a previous existence. In his dialogue *Meno*, Plato pictures a simple, uneducated slave-boy being interrogated by Socrates. With a

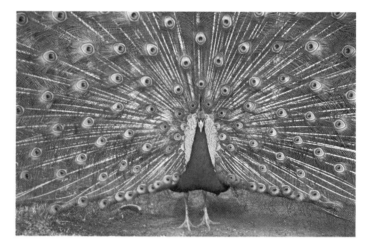

Reacting appropriately to stereotyped situations: a male peacock displays its tail feathers.

judicious choice of questions, Socrates drags out of him an account of the fundamental theorems of geometry. True knowledge, Plato argues, must be within us all, and learning consists solely of discovering what we already know.

It is true that the genetically programmed wiring of the brain restricts the way in which each animal can act, and even provides a vast repertoire of inherited automatic reflexes that allow it, without previous personal experience, to react appropriately to certain stereotyped situations that it might encounter. Built-in reflexes *are* the inherent knowledge of Plato; they are the behavioural reflections of genetic memories about the experiences of earlier brains. To the extent that inherent reflexes are based on patterns of connections in the brain, programmed by the DNA of the genes, it is correct to say that this small component of mental memory is coded in a chemical form. But it is inconceivable that the empirical experience of each individual animal is actually represented by the synthesis of molecules. The expression of even innate reflexes requires the construction of nerve pathways that guarantee the appropriate response to the particular stimulus. The formation of personal memories must surely involve a similar transformation in the connectivity of the brain.

112

It is not surprising then to discover that the brains of learning animals synthesize more R N A and protein, and that drugs that prevent such synthesis also block the ability to learn. Increased metabolic activity and changes in the efficiency of contacts between the nerve cells in any circuit must both involve the synthesis of protein. But, although the protein produced is derived ultimately

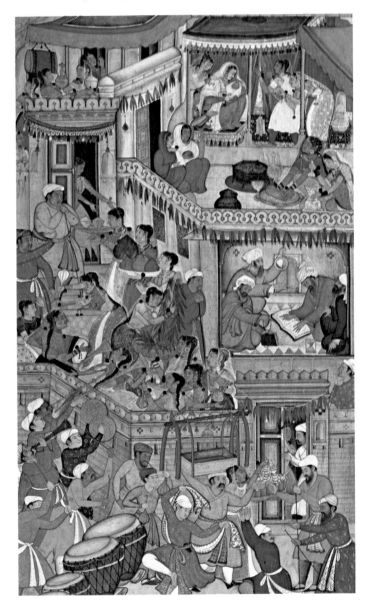

To anticipate the future is the ultimate goal. At the birth of Murrad, second son of the Moghul emperor Akbar, in 1570, the casting of an astrological chart was a natural part of the celebrations. Indian miniature (c. 1590) by Bhura.

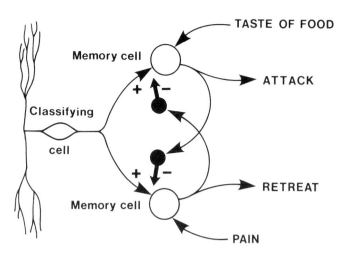

Simple pre-existing networks of nerve cells can be made to 'learn' as long as they contain 'modifiable synapses' – junctions that can be strengthened or weakened on the basis of the success or failure of the animal's preceding response. J. Z. Young designed this simple memory model, called the 'mnemon', to explain discrimination learning in an octopus. The animal can look at a simple visual pattern and learn to approach it in order to obtain food, or to retreat from it to avoid an electric shock. This model is partly based on known connections in the octopus' brain. Imagine groups of 'classifying cells' that detect the shapes of patterns in front of the eyes. These cells might, through their connections on to other, so-called 'memory cells', set off an attack or a retreat. The presence of food could increase the chance of an attack, and pain could make retreat more likely. When either pathway is active it turns off the alternative one by inhibiting the other memory cells, via small inhibitory neurons, drawn as filled circles. Learning, according to J. Z. Young's scheme, could take place by the strengthening of the synaptic contacts on these small inhibitory cells, so that whenever one pathway has been employed on several occasions, the alternative pathway would be permanently inhibited. Thus a certain visual signal would come to evoke a certain response.

from messages in the genetic DNA, it is not *that* code that contains the new, personal memory. The resulting change in the pattern of nerve connections *is* the memory. What the chromosomes must store is the instruction needed to allow any circuit to change depending on its own activity, without specifying in advance which circuit will be involved. The ultimate chemical contribution to mental memory is, then, the genetically-programmed ability to learn.

The emergence of the capacity to learn is the triumph of evolution. Its first appearance must have been, quite simply, a transcendent step in the development of animal life, for learning frees the individual from the chains of his own double helix. It is the predictive power of learning and memory that give them such immense survival value. A primary requirement of any animal is that it should be able to anticipate changes in its environment. Inherited reflexes contain a static description of the events of high probability in the past experience of the species, but learning allows each animal to add a stock of personal secrets to its description of the probabilities of the world.

To anticipate the future is the ultimate goal of the evolution of the nervous system. But since it works inductively, the brain can only base its predictions on

114

probabilities drawn from the past. True clairvoyance – the mythical power of the soothsayer to predict future events without statistical qualification – would be so immensely valuable to an animal that its natural selection by evolutionary pressure would have been explosive. If any species had had genuine second sight, not only would it necessarily have spread like a flood through the gene pool, but also that species would rule the world. For this reason alone the biologist must regard with extreme suspicion the claim that some individuals have extra-sensory perception or true clairvoyance. And yet we do owe a good deal of our own biological superiority to our ability to plan for the future. There is no doubt that the evolution of intelligence has involved a gradually increasing power of prediction.

In the back-to-front world that Alice found behind the Looking Glass, the White Queen actually *lived* in

The histories of astrology and astronomy are intimately entwined. Ptolemy, a careful astronomer, whose model of the universe was dogma throughout the Middle Ages, was fascinated by the possibility of prediction of future events. Perhaps the discovery of the inevitable progression of the stars led to the idea that events on earth are predestined and bound to the motion of the heavens. On the left is a Roman sculpture of Jupiter in a zodiac circle (probably second century). On the right is an astrolabe (probably sixteenth century) by Arssenius; it was used to measure the positions of planets and stars for navigational purposes – true prediction based on the pattern of heavenly bodies.

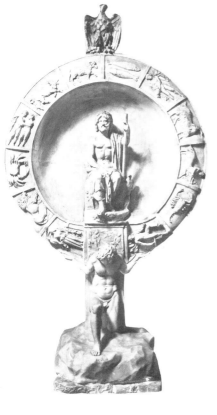

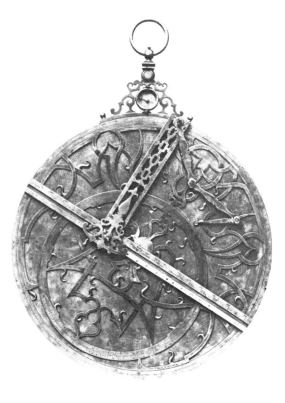

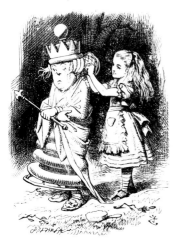

Alice and the White Queen: illustration by Sir John Tenniel for the first edition of Lewis Carroll's Through the Looking Glass, *1896.*

reverse. 'There's one great advantage in it', she said, 'that one's memory works both ways.'

Alice remarked: 'I'm sure *mine* only works one way. I can't remember things before they happen', to which the White Queen replied: 'It's a poor sort of memory that only works backwards.'

And so it is. Our memory is not quite the kind of bizarre predictor of the future that made the White Queen scream *before* her finger was pricked, but the biological (if not the aesthetic) value of remembering is not that it allows one to reminisce about the past, but that it permits one to calculate coldly about the unknown future.

Just as individual memory has partly released each animal from the immediate restrictions of the genetic code, so the sharing of learned ideas by social animals has added an entirely new dimension to the progress of evolution. The spread of ideas through social groups of animals, which is so well developed in the primates, and especially in man, allows the experience of the individual to become reflected in the behaviour of other members of the same social group, even those in later generations. This is truly the social inheritance of culturally acquired characteristics.

In 1953, on the Japanese island of Koshima, a female macaque monkey called Imo, a genius amongst monkeys, invented a method for cleaning unpalatable sand from the sweet potatoes that the group of scientists observing the monkeys had been scattering on the beach since the previous year. She dipped each potato into the water of a brook with one hand and brushed away the sand with the other. During the following two years this habit of washing potatoes spread to 90 per cent of the members of Imo's troop: only the youngest infants did not know it, and the oldest males steadfastly refused to adopt it.

In 1955 Imo made an even more remarkable discovery. The biologists had also been spreading wheat on the beach for the monkeys; but picking it, grain by grain, from the sand was a tedious business. Imo invented a method of sifting the wheat by flotation. She threw handfuls of it into the sea; the sand sank and she skimmed the grains from the surface. Again, within a few years this difficult skill had been mastered by a majority of the juvenile monkeys.

By the sharing of ideas, animals, and most especially humans, pool the ability of their group. The pinnacles of intelligence are exploited by the entire society. In human culture, this has led to the emergence of a kind of communal intellect – the Collective Mind of man – that has pushed forward his biological progress at a prodigious rate. At first the cultural transmission of human ideas must have been by imitation or demonstration, as it is amongst monkeys, and later by word of mouth. Such methods of transfer are subject to the opportunity for progressive distortion like that which characterizes the spreading of a rumour. And hence all the conditions would exist for a kind of evolution of ideas. The variability, which genetic mutation gives in Darwinian evolution, would be provided by the regular contribution of individual new ideas and their distortion in cultural

Distortion of images during copying and re-copying is seen in these sets of ancient British coins, based on the original Greek models shown at the left.

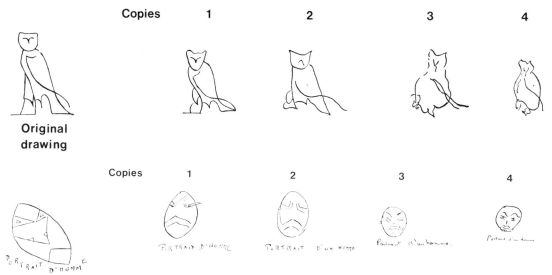

| Copies | 1 | 2 | 3 | 4 |

Original drawing

| Copies | 1 | 2 | 3 | 4 |

Original drawing

Sir Frederic Bartlett (1886–1969), first Professor of Experimental Psychology in Cambridge, made a fascinating study of remembering, and became interested in the social transmission of information. He performed experiments on the sequential distortion of messages as they were transmitted by voice or by drawing from one individual to another. In each series illustrated here, the first observer saw the original drawings (a hieroglyphic owl or a mask-like portrait). He then reproduced it from memory and his drawing was shown to the next person in the series, who again drew from memory what he had seen, and so on. The images were gradually transformed.

transfer. The natural selection of these ideas would be made on the basis of their utility; in general, useful ideas would survive because they would propagate themselves, just as an adaptive genetic mutation flourishes.

In effect, the evolution of ideas in the Collective Mind of man has virtually brought true natural selection to a halt. The ability of man to manipulate and plunder his environment has steadily grown, at the same time that medical skill has almost vanquished the forces that put pressure on the biologically undesirable elements of his genetic stock. Many biologists, including Jacques Monod, the French Nobel prize winner, have expressed their fears at the dilution in quality of the human gene pool. But that is not all we have to fear. The present status of humanity is in fact a stalemate between the forces of conventional evolution, which threaten to punish us for breaking beyond the bounds of our biological rights, and our Collective Mind, which battles to preserve our present status. What we should be most afraid of, perhaps, is the fact that, since the invention of printing, magnetic tape and computer cards, the Collective Mind

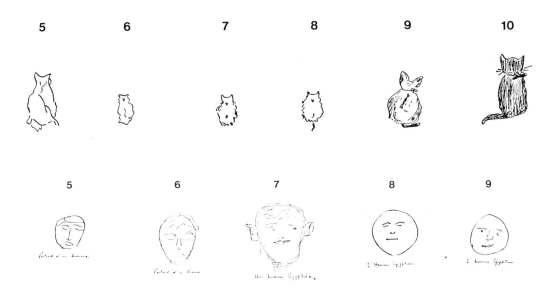

has lost the vital ability to *forget*. A principal task for us lies in the organization of knowledge for ready access. This problem is nowhere more acute than in science itself, where the sheer accumulation of facts threatens to impede rather than to assist the progress of new ideas.

Already the technology that supports everyday life in the developed world has become so complex that no single mind can understand it. Man might not go out with a bang of his own creation, nor freeze his race to death by stealing the energy resources of the earth. He might merely drown himself in a flood of information; society could collapse because it no longer comprehends its own cultural inheritance.

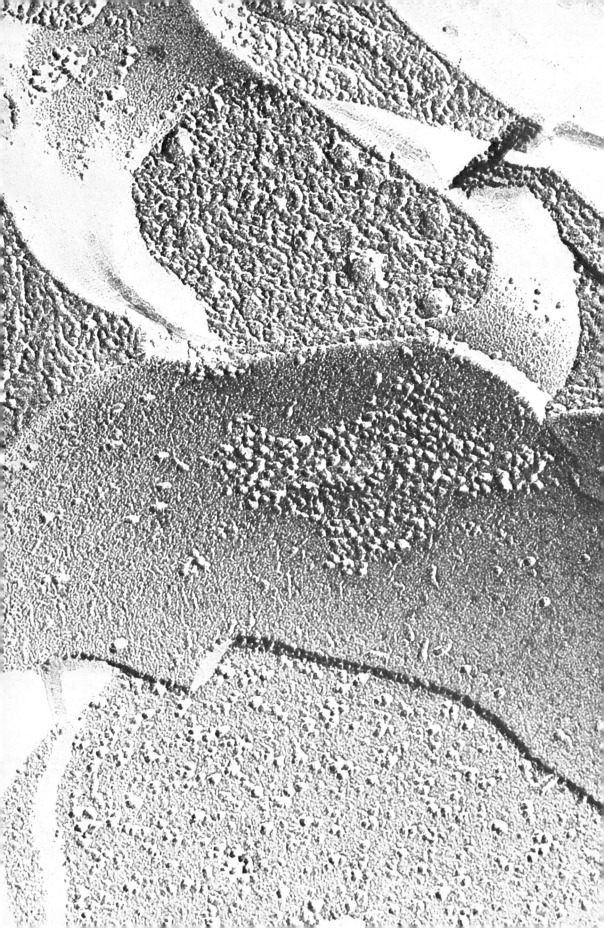

*A new anatomical technique –
freeze-fracture – allows the synapse
itself to be split open and the
surfaces of the nerve terminal and
dendrite or cell body to be inspected.
A tiny sample of brain tissue is very
rapidly frozen (in about
a second) and then broken. The
material tends to split along lines of
weakness, such as the synaptic gaps
between terminal membranes and
post-synaptic membranes. The
fractured surface is then covered with
a thin film of platinum and carbon,
which is viewed in the
electron microscope. This
freeze-fracture micrograph, made by
Konrad Akert and his colleagues in
Zürich, is of neurons in the optic
tectum (the sub-cortical visual area)
of the pigeon's brain, and it is
magnified about 175,000 times. The
flat area in the middle is probably
the synaptic surface of a nerve cell,
where a terminal has been broken
away. The cluster of particles on
the membrane surface may be
specialized 'receptor' molecules,
thought to be stimulated by the
transmitter substance which is
released by the terminal and which
diffuses across the minute synaptic
gap. Conceivably, the strengthening
of synapses during learning could
involve an increase in the density of
these receptor molecules or a change
in their properties.*

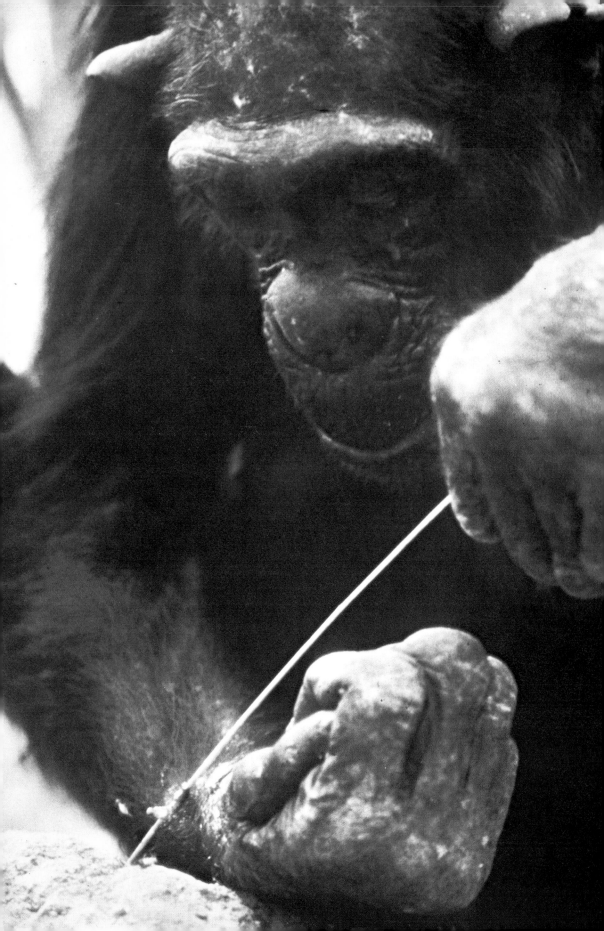

5 A burning fire

Eyesight and speech they wrought
  For the veil of the soul therein,
A time for labour and thought,
  A time to serve and to sin;
They gave him light in his ways,
  And love, and a space for delight,
And beauty and length of days,
  And night, and sleep in the night.
His speech is a burning fire;
  With his lips he travaileth;
In his heart is a blind desire;
  In his eyes foreknowledge of death;
He weaves, and is clothed with derision;
  Sows, and he shall not reap;
His life is a watch or a vision
  Between a sleep and a sleep.
  A. C. Swinburne (1837–1909), *Atalanta in Calydon*

A few years ago, in the small town of Norman, Oklahoma, a reporter from the *New York Times* had a brief conversation with a little girl called Lucy.

He held up a key and asked, 'What's this?'

'Key', Lucy replied.

Then he picked up a comb; 'What's this?'

'Comb', answered Lucy, as she took it from his hands and proceeded to comb his hair. She stopped.

'Comb me', she pleaded.

'O.K.', he said, and combed her.

'Lucy, you want to go outside?', he suggested.

123

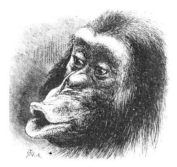

Speaking is something that chimpanzees simply cannot do. This drawing, from Darwin's The Expression of the Emotions in Man and Animals *(1872), shows a disappointed and sulky chimpanzee emitting part of its limited vocal repertoire.*

She thought for a while and replied, 'Outside, no. Want food; apple.'

'I have no food', he apologized, 'Sorry.'

A singularly unremarkable dialogue, one might think; indeed, the girl seemed rather backward in her grammar. But there again she had been separated from her mother just four days after she was born in 1966, and was brought up by foster parents. And the conversation was not *spoken*; it was conducted with a series of hand movements, in American Sign Language for the deaf. Lucy is not deaf, however; she is a chimpanzee. And her foster parents were human. She is a member of a small and elite group of apes who are, unknowingly, excavating the foundations on which man has built the myth of his biological uniqueness.

The attempt to teach language to apes has a history of at least fifty years, but early efforts foundered because they sought to persuade chimpanzees to do something that they simply cannot do – to speak. Most of these animals were reared alongside the experimenters' own babies, and they proved more than a match for their human infant companions, in both agility and intellect, until the baby 'naked apes' began to speak. Then, apparently repeating the evolutionary history of man, the human infants soon outstripped their simian colleagues. The failure of chimpanzees to talk seemed to betray a fundamental barrier in their ability to think, and to bestow a special status on the intelligence of man.

According to René Descartes, what man has, besides an animal's clockwork brain, is a rational soul. And a distinguishing feature of that rational soul is the capacity for *propositional* speech, the synthesis of words into statements that, by their form, give extra meaning to those words. Descartes' supreme role for language is echoed in the opinion of successive philosophers and biologists who searched for special characteristics that might explain man's phenomenal cultural progress.

The more that ethologists have learned about the apes, however, the shorter has become the list of supposedly unique human attributes. The use of tools and the solution of problems by insight can no longer be considered as defining features of man. Virtually the only things that can be defended as uniquely human traits are his continuous sexual appetite, his formal taboo on incest, and his language. 'All of man's unique social behaviour,' writes the biologist Edward Wilson, 'pivots on his use of language, which is itself unique.' Algernon Swinburne called human speech 'a burning fire', and there can be no doubt that the use of language was just as important in human evolution as the discovery of flame itself. But now the experiments with American Sign Language threaten to force man to share this ultimate cultural crown with the apes.

Two American psychologists, Allen and Beatrice Gardner, started the project, in Nevada, in 1966. The

At the Institute of Primate Studies, Norman, Oklahoma, where Washoe and Lucy now live, a number of other chimpanzees are being taught American Sign Language. They use it to communicate amongst themselves, and it is thought that they might teach it to their offspring. Here two young male chimpanzees, Ally and Bruno, give the gesture for 'listen', as their human colleague points to his watch.

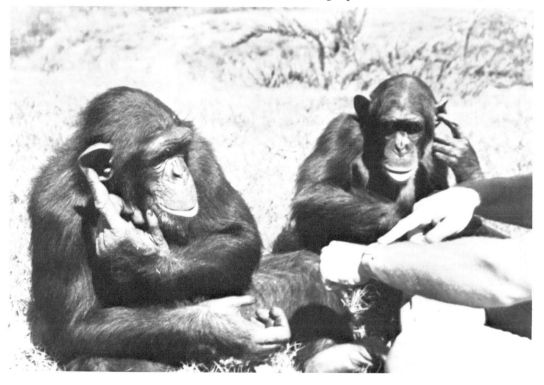

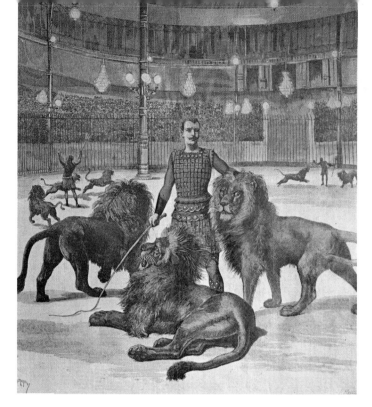

Is language, as B. F. Skinner argues, essentially the learning of associations, like the operant conditioning of circus animals; or is it dependent on some uniquely human, innate capacity? 'Neron à l'Hippodrome', circus poster, 1894.

first scholar in their academy for apes was a one-year-old chimpanzee called Washoe, whom they kept in a luxurious trailer home, surrounded by obsequious attendants who constantly talked to her and to each other in hand language. By the age of five, Washoe had learned the gestural signs for nearly 200 words, including adjectives and verbs as well as nouns. This in itself was not surprising, for learning to make a certain movement of the arms in order to receive a desired object is, in principle, no more of an achievement than learning to beg or jump through a hoop for a piece of food. Words alone do not make propositional speech. Were the words made into the flesh of a genuine language? Did Washoe manipulate her manual lexicon within the framework of a true grammar? That question is still being fiercely contested amongst professional linguists, but I think that the evidence is overwhelming that Washoe has acquired a language – primitive, but not fundamentally different from our own.

First, consider the nature of words themselves. Each

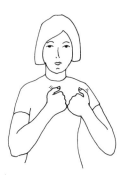

1916

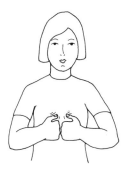

PRESENT

During the past sixty years American Sign Language has gradually changed, perhaps in a manner analogous to the evolution of spoken language. Films taken in 1913 show that the old sign for 'sweetheart' was very iconic, the hands being placed over the left side of the chest in the shape of a heart. The present-day sign is made in the centre of the body and is much more abstract. In the same way, very early spoken language may have contained a much greater fraction of onomatopoeia. From a study by Edward Klima and Ursula Bellugi.

Consider the nature of words. Text ▶ of the psalm 'Dominus dixit Domino' from the Ormesby Psalter, Bodleian Library, Oxford (Ms Douce 366, F. 146 verso).

spoken language consists of a relatively small number of distinguishable sounds called *phonemes* – usually about 40 or 50 of them – like the 'ch' and the 'p' in 'chimpanzee'. The first thing that a legitimate language must do is to use units like phonemes in combination to generate a potentially infinite variety of words; there are about 150,000 words in English. There is no certain evidence at the moment that any natural animal communication systems – bird songs, insect dances or the individual smells of mammals, for instance – have the richness created by arbitrarily combining elementary signals into a multitude of meanings.

Now Washoe, and Lucy, the chimpanzees who can talk with their hands, were never *expected* to create their own meaningful gestures from a combination of meaningless fragments of movement, any more than a child learns phonemes and then synthesizes words. And yet these chimpanzees *have* spontaneously invented a few

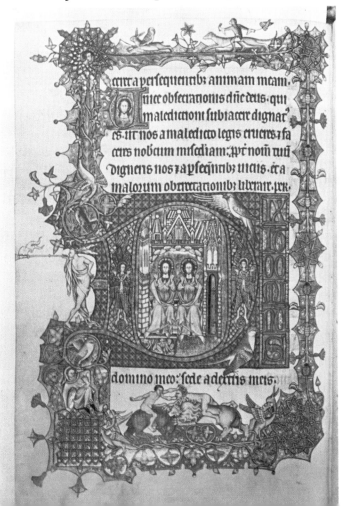

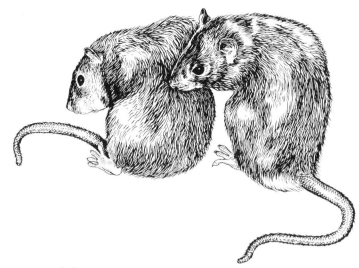

'Allogrooming', the grooming of one animal by another, is a common form of social communication in rodents. Here a male wild rat grooms a male newcomer to his cage, as a sign of conciliation. (From Barnett, 1975).

signs of their own, suggesting that they understand the principle of combining 'gestural phonemes'. Washoe, for example, signalled for her bib by drawing its outline on her chest. This is, in fact the correct sign for 'bib' in American Sign Language, though the Gardners did not know it at the time. Lucy also uses a kind of gestural onomatopoeia in her invented word for the halter that she has to wear during walks: she mimes the act of putting on the leash, and often precedes it by the gesture for 'dirty', just to indicate her disgust at having to wear it.

Even more interesting is the way in which Washoe, Lucy, and the others couple their limited stocks of words together to manufacture new ones. According to Lucy, a watermelon is a 'drink-fruit' or a 'candy-drink' and a strong radish is 'cry-hurt-food'. And even though she has been taught a single gesture for 'refrigerator', Washoe prefers to call it an 'open-food-drink'. Is this true linguistic resourcefulness, approaching the human use of language to classify phenomena and hence to comprehend the world? Perhaps. It is certainly more than the pairing of a response with an object or picture.

But sceptics might still say that these apes do no more than perform associations like Pavlov's dogs or Skinner's

Early Egyptian picture writing was essentially a set of stylized drawings telling a story. Narmer Palette, Upper Egypt, c. 3200 B.C. First dynasty.

The later hieroglyphic style was much more abstract, but still contained pictorial elements. A stele from the tomb of Huntnu, eleventh dynasty, 2134–2000 B.C.

129

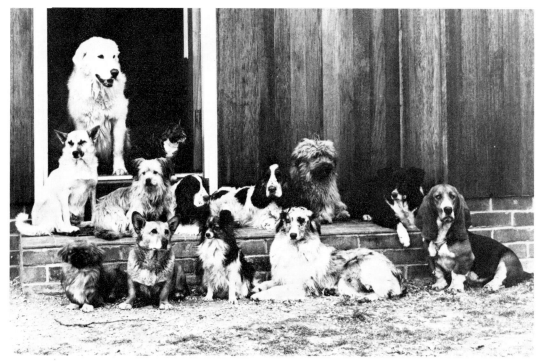

Is it linguistic thought that enables us instantly to spot the odd-animal-out?

rats. For a man, a word is much more than a label attached to a particular action or thing. It is the product of a cognitive analysis in which things are recognized as members of classes. Think how difficult it would be to explain to a visitor from space just why four-legged animals that bark, that have fur and that wag their tails, are usually called 'dogs', and then why it is that not all animals we call dogs have exactly the same kind of fur, why some dogs do *not* bark and why others have *no* tails. Each time that we say 'I see a dog', we are, in a sense, performing an exercise in logic of staggering complexity; the immediate characteristics of the object we see are checked against the salient common features of all previously encountered dogs in our internal model of 'dogginess'. Words, then, are general postulates derived through specific examples – they are the result of powerful *inductive* reasoning. But they have *deductive* consequences with predictive force. Thus they are used to classify objects that have never been experienced before

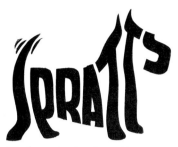

Words are theories about objects.
Trade name for pet food.

and to deduce the expected properties and actions of those objects. Suppose that we see an entirely new breed of animal, and decide from its appearance that it is a 'dog'. By fitting it into a general class, we can immediately forecast what its behaviour is likely to be.

Just as the deductive consequences of a scientific hypothesis predict the outcome of particular experiments, so words are theories about objects. The capacity to use words to classify, and hence to prophesy, must have been of immense value in man's struggle to understand and ultimately to control his environment. Some would say that language has actually formed the way in which we think, and that linguistic classification is the basis of a uniquely human mode of thought. As a little girl once said to Graham Wallas, the author of *The Art of Thought*, 'How can I know what I think till I see what I say?'

Perhaps animals cannot generalize from experiences into concepts, because they lack the advantage of linguistically moulded thought. The seekers-after-uniqueness for man would cherish this notion, for it would imply that not only speech, but also the superior mode of thinking behind it, are man's alone.

Take the case of another chimpanzee, Rafael by name, who was being studied by Pavlov's group of research workers. Rafael had learned to use a jar of water, drawn from a tap in a barrel, to extinguish a burning wick that blocked his way to food. He could also use a bamboo pole as a bridge to cross from one raft, floating on a lake, to another one nearby. One sweltering summer's day, Rafael, watched by a team of scientists, sat on a raft cooling himself by collecting water from the lake with his hand and pouring it over his head. One of the experimenters rowed across to Rafael's raft, put some fruit at one end and a burning wick to block Rafael's way. On a neighbouring raft stood the familiar water barrel. Rafael surveyed the scene; suddenly, in a flash of

131

inspiration, he threw his bamboo pole across to the other raft, struggled over it, filled his jar from the tap in the barrel, climbed back, put out the fire and swallowed the fruit! But this pinnacle of insight was an abyss of stupidity. Any person would have doused the fire with the same source of water that Rafael had been using to soak himself. But to Rafael they were not the same thing; he seemed to have no general concept of 'water'. He had no internal word for it.

On the other hand, Washoe and friends *have* passed this test of generalization. Washoe used the sign 'dog' for dogs in *pictures* as well as real ones. She signalled 'flower' to indicate anything that smelled strongly, like a tobacco pouch or menthol ointment, and later corrected this faulty generalization by learning a different sign for 'smell'; then she only used 'flower' to mean a blossom. And though she learned the gesture meaning 'open' for the door of her home, she soon applied it to boxes and bottles as well.

Even with words, even with generalization, no language is a language with words alone. The semantics of a statement – its meaning – depends on the syntax of its structure. Even ten words could make a language, but without grammar they would be nothing but an impoverished dictionary. Only by the order and relationships of words in sentences can we free our utterances from the prison of the present moment and talk of the past or the future. The property of *displacement* – communicating events that are remote in time or place – is fundamental to true language; and displacement in language rests on the extra dimension that grammar gives to words.

It is true that some of the acts of natural animal communication do have the rudiments of displacement. The frenzied kissing ceremony of a pack of African wild dogs, before it starts to hunt, is an emotional discussion about future events. Edward Wilson translates their

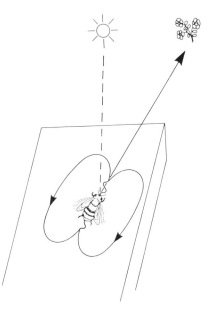

The dance of the honey bee. The bee walks in a figure-of-eight pattern; the central section consists of a waggling run, whose direction points to the source of nectar, relative to the sun. The length of the waggle-run specifies the distance of the food, with an operational accuracy of about 20 per cent.

imagined conversation: 'I submerge my identity ... I will do my share of the hunting. I will share in the feeding. Let's go! Let's go!' Similarly, the extraordinary waggle dance of a honey bee communicates the distance and direction of a remote source of nectar to her fellow workers. In the dance, which was deciphered by Karl von Frisch, the bee runs forward, violently shaking her abdomen. The length of the run represents the distance of the food source and the direction of the dance points towards it, using the sun as the reference in space. It is, in fact, a graphical representation of the flight pattern needed to reach the food.

But these fragments of displacement in animal communication are still merely stereotyped expressions of the animals' immediate needs. They are almost trivial compared with the power of human language to lift man out of the grip of his emotions, to let him conjecture, plan and explain.

Again, as with words, the structure of grammar reveals the machinery of the human mind – the analysis of events into sequences of actions. Indeed, one of the major tenets of modern linguistics is that most of the

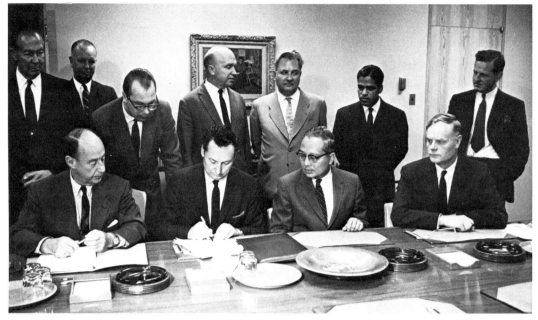

The power of human language to lift man out of the grip of his emotions. Nikolai Federenko, Sir Patrick Dean and Adlai Stevenson sign the partial Test Ban Treaty, under the eye of U Thant, at the United Nations Building, New York, 15 October 1963.

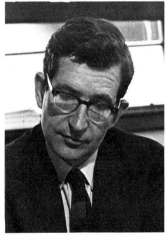

Noam Chomsky.

rules of grammar operate independently of meaning. In his revolutionary theory of syntax, Noam Chomsky claimed that people have within them an innate, universal system of syntax which makes them competent to learn to understand and to generate speech. This knowledge is the prerequisite for any human language. It comprises the laws that govern the formation of elementary sentences; these 'deep structures' are propositional descriptions, which are transformed into the permissible utterances of a particular language by a set of grammatical rules. As the Duchess in Wonderland said to Alice: 'Take care of the sense and the sounds will take care of themselves.'!

The following sentence recently opened an important review article in the scientific journal *Nature*: '... hadrons consist of quarks bound by vector gluons'.

The statement is clearly grammatical; it obeys the rules of English sentence structure. But it is quite meaningless without knowledge of the vocabulary of modern particle physics. Chomsky himself uses the semantically nonsensical but syntactically perfect sen-

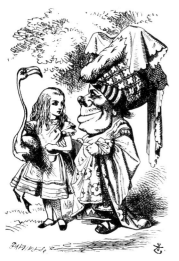

'The sounds will take care of themselves'. Alice and the Duchess, from Lewis Carroll's Alice's Adventures in Wonderland, 1896.

tence, 'Colourless green ideas sleep furiously' to illustrate the concept that much of grammatical structure is independent of meaning. Grammar can be more precisely formulated than meaning.

It is here, at the question of grammar, that the interpretation of Washoe's achievements becomes most controversial. In 1969 the Gardners wrote:

'From the time she had eight or ten signs in her repertoire, Washoe began to use them in strings of two or more . . . we made no deliberate effort to elicit combinations other than by our habitual use of strings of signs. Some of the combined forms that Washoe has used may have been imitative, but many have been inventions of her own.'

To begin with most of Washoe's 'sentences' consisted of only a pair of signs, but even these two-word phrases seemed to have much the same kind of elementary grammar that children use when they first combine pairs of words; Washoe was less than two years old at the time – just about the age when children first add words together. The terse phrases that human infants utter in this first stage of language have a strange 'telegraphic' style, which conveys meaning but may have only a very primitive syntax of its own: 'big train', 'walk street' and 'hit ball' are good examples. And Washoe's first combinations were very similar: 'hurry open', 'more tickle' and 'Roger come'.

In children's speech, the cultural individuality of the native language begins to emerge when three words are first put together. And just ten months after she joined Allen and Beatrice Gardner, Washoe started combining three or more signs. At first she tended to put both subject and object before the verb, as in 'Roger Washoe tickle', and made other mixtures that would be errors in word order in English, like 'You out go'. But her manual conversations have gradually settled into a pat-

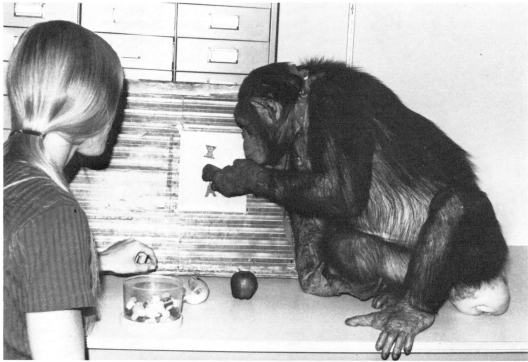

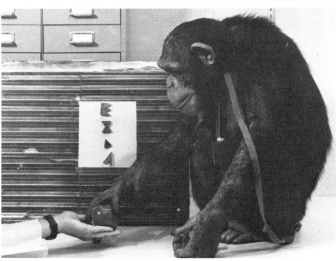

In California, David Premack has used a somewhat different approach in his study of the capacity for language in apes. He and his colleagues teach chimpanzees to communicate by 'writing' messages with abstract metal symbols stuck on a magnetized board. Chimpanzees can learn such concepts as 'same' and 'different', the naming of colours and the 'if . . . then' construction. Here a six-year-old African-born chimpanzee, Elizabeth, writes the sentence 'Elizabeth give apple Amy' (the triangle shape means 'apple') and then proceeds to carry out the action. She wears a necklace, with the symbol for her own name strung on it.

tern rather like that of English, the style used by her trainers. She nearly always puts the subject before the verb, and is quite capable of detecting differences in meaning from changes in order, such as 'You tickle me' and 'Me tickle you'. In short, Washoe and her friends are slowly but surely tracing the path that leads to real language. If propositional language is the qualification needed for membership in humanity, then Washoe seems to be eligible, at least as much as a two-year-old child!

What should we make, then, of Chomsky's suggestion that the formal properties of language are not only unique to man but are innately determined – a behavioural expression of a genetically inherited structure in the brain? Is a baby, as Ronald Knox would have us believe, 'a loud noise at one end and no sense of responsibility at the other'? Or is it an articulate human creature, struggling to escape from a speechless skin? Chomsky points out that children make grammatically sensible errors, such as 'two sheeps' and 'Mummy sitted', showing that they apply syntactical rules and do not simply learn every utterance individually. And he thinks that the complexity of grammar (which seems to defy mere learning), and the fact that all languages may have a common 'deep structure', point to an inherited basis. However, there is no *a priori* reason why learning should not produce organization in the brain as complex as the mechanism of inheritance. And the common 'deep structure' of languages may not necessarily reflect an identical origin in human genes. It could be that the problem of communicating propositional thoughts is so elaborate that only *one* solution is possible, and that it has been reached independently, through cultural transmission and enrichment, in all societies. To take a biological analogy, the eye of a mammal like man, and of a cephalopod like an octopus, look virtually identical. In almost every respect they resemble each other very closely. Yet, in evolutionary terms, they do not have the same origins. They are constructed in quite different ways within the developing embryo, and they must each have evolved as completely independent, but uncannily similar, solutions to the problem of seeing, through a

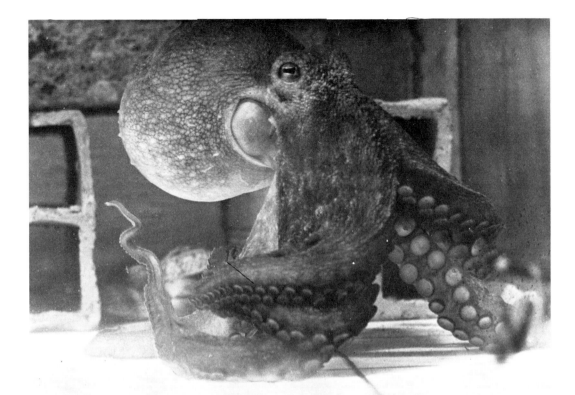

The cephalopod eye is remarkably like the mammalian eye (and even more like that of a fish) although its evolutionary origins are quite different. An octopus advances on its prey. The horizontal, slit-shaped pupil can be seen in the close-up of the eye.

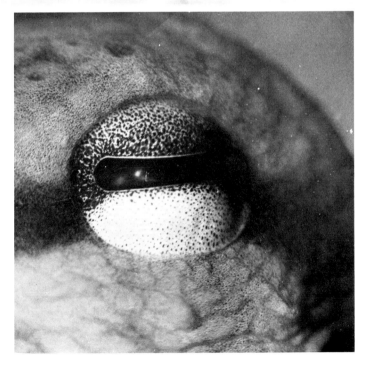

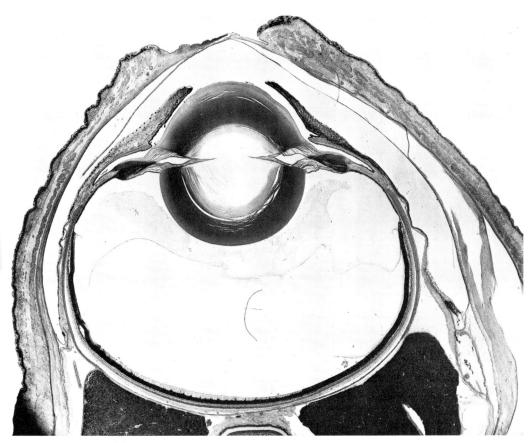

Above is a cross-section of the octopus eye, photographed by J. Z. Young. The huge spherical lens, of great power, is clearly visible, with the iris lying on its upper surface. Below is Descartes' diagram of a similar cross-section through the mammalian eye, from La Dioptrique, 1637. L is the lens, and H the 'optic disc', where nerve fibres leave the eye to form the optic nerve (Z).

The two types of eye, though superficially similar to each other, have quite different retinal organization. The cephalopod retina has its photoreceptors pointing out towards the centre of the eye, and contains no other types of neuron. The mammalian eye has layers of nerve cells lying on top of its receptors, which actually point backwards; light must pass through all the cell layers to reach the rods and cones. These differences betray the different origins of the two kinds of eye.

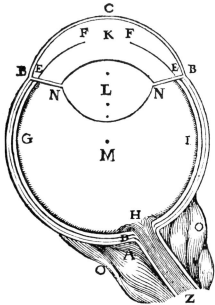

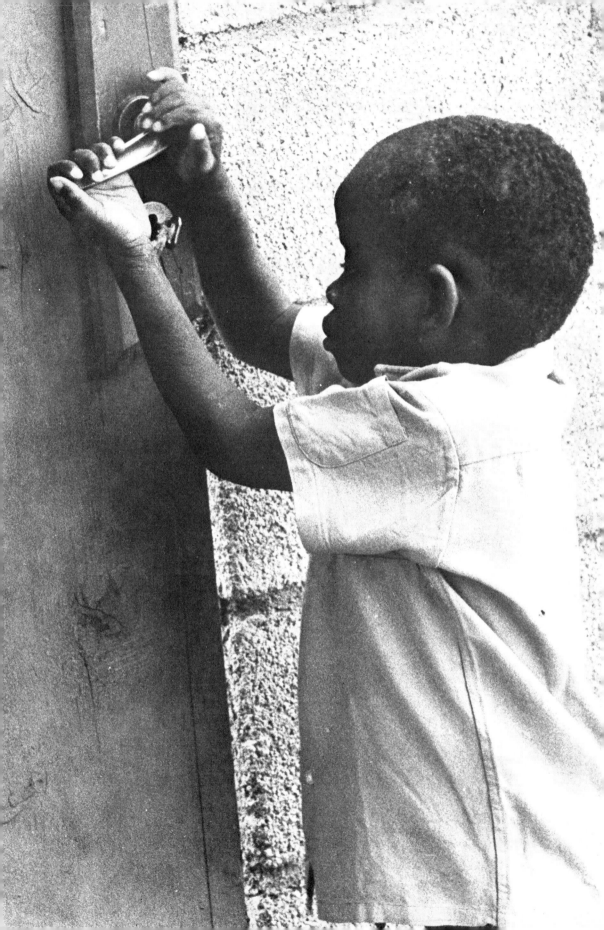

process known as evolutionary convergence. One could argue that the task of talking, like seeing, is so demanding that the same single solution may have been arrived at by many separate *cultural* evolutions.

It is true that any child can learn any tongue, as long as he starts early enough. But it is almost certain that children would develop no language at all without continuous and lengthy lessons from an expert. There is, in fact, a *critical period* during which an infant's developing brain is able to master, by experience, the skill of talking. If he has no contact with speaking people before the age of about seven years old, a child will have the greatest difficulty in learning language later on. In classical Imperial Japan, an infant was not considered to be human until it was seven years old and could be abandoned by its parents, with impenitence and without fear of retribution. How remarkably Cartesian this custom seems: Not until a child had passed through the critical time for acquisition of language was it truly a human being.

Again, damage to the brain almost never causes irreversible loss of language in a child still within the critical age. But, sadly, irremediable loss *is* a common consequence of brain injury in adults. The clinical study of language began in earnest with a remarkable piece of scientific prediction. At a stormy meeting of the Société d'Anthropologie in Paris, on 4 April 1861, Simon Auburtin, the son-in-law of a once famous expert in phrenology, Jean-Baptiste Bouillaud, announced his conviction that the power of speech is localized in the frontal lobes of the cerebral hemispheres. His own clinical evidence was slight, but he predicted that any patient who had lost the power of speech though not the ability to understand it would be found, if his brain were examined, to have damage or degeneration in the frontal lobes. The secretary of the meeting was a surgeon, Pierre-Paul Broca, and just a few days later he came

This boy, called Johann by nurses at the orphanage in Burundi where he lives, was discovered about four years ago amongst a group of apes by peasant farmers near Rumonge on the shores of Lake Tanganyika. He was about four years old at the time of his capture and it is conceivable that he had been abandoned in 1972 during warfare in that area between the Watusi and the Hudu tribes; he may have been living wild, perhaps with the apes. He was totally naked and quite hairy, and he mainly walked on all fours. He has not spoken a word since he was caught but he communicates with facial expressions and violent gesticulation. He is now seven or eight years old and is approaching the end of the sensitive period for the acquisition of verbal language. Interestingly, the use of his hands is also poorly developed. Here he struggles to open a door.

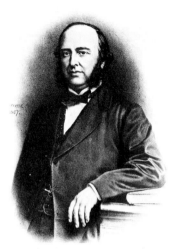

Pierre-Paul Broca (1824–1880).

across a patient who for years had suffered from weakness in the right side of his body and a virtually total inability to speak. Almost the only sound that he could utter was 'Tan' and this has become his name in the annals of medical history. Tan died on 17 April 1861, and Broca immediately carried out a post mortem examination. The very next day, he reported the result to the Société d'Anthropologie. Auburtin's premonition was substantiated: the frontal lobes of Tan's brain had degenerated severely.

Two years later Broca had seen several more cases and he wrote: 'Here are eight instances in which the injury was in the posterior third of the third frontal convolution. This number seems to me to be sufficient to give strong presumptions. And the most remarkable thing is that in all the patients the injury was on the left side. I do not dare draw conclusions from this. I await new facts.'

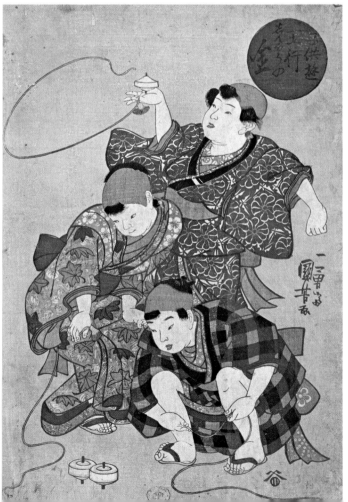

Children in Imperial Japan. 'Playing with tops' by Ichiyusai Kuniyoshi (1797–1861), Utagawa School, late Edo Era.

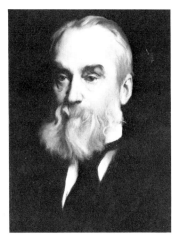

John Hughlings Jackson (1835–1911).

The conclusion that Broca did not dare to draw is the one that is now widely accepted: the mental mechanism for speech is nearly always localized on the left side of the brain. Now there had been speculation even in ancient times that *movement* in one half of the body is controlled by the opposite half of the brain. Tan's right-sided muscular weakness was due to the degeneration that affected the motor area in his left frontal lobe. The speech area, which now bears Broca's name, is close by, but separate from the part of the motor cortex that controls movements of the tongue and larynx.

The British neurologist John Hughlings Jackson pointed out that speech could suffer without any paralysis of the tongue, lips or palate, and indeed that some aspects of speech could be lost without others. He described the case of the daughter of his driver who was taking him to school when he was a boy. She suddenly became almost dumb during the journey and they returned home. Hughlings Jackson wrote:

'I remember being struck by a self-contradictory expression made use of by the patient. She said, "I can't talk" . . . She gradually lost speech altogether . . . For three weeks she did not utter a word, but was apparently conscious . . . The first word she ever uttered was in reply to a question – addressed to her in order to get her to talk – she said "waistcoat". It had no bearing on the question.'

With Broca's area damaged, what speech remains is reduced to a curt, telegraphic style rather like the first phrases of children. It is laborious and taxing and sometimes the words just cannot come. Another British neurologist, Sir Henry Head, working after the turn of the century, described such a patient who could understand most questions and if his answer were 'Yes', could say so; but he could never say 'No'. Instead he would simply say 'Damn!'.

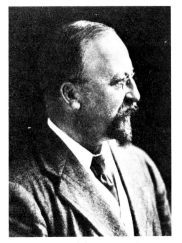

Sir Henry Head (1861–1940).

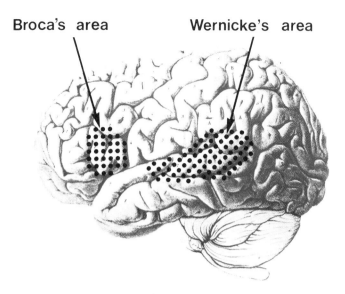

Broca's area **Wernicke's area**

The positions of Broca's and Wernicke's areas are superimposed on Gratiolet's (1854) diagram of the left side of the brain.

In 1874, Karl Wernicke discovered that damage further back in the left cerebral hemisphere, mainly in the temporal lobe, can cause a loss in the understanding of the spoken and written word, with less disturbance of speech itself. This region of the brain, now known as Wernicke's area, lies close to the auditory cortex, which analyses sound. In the majority of people this region is actually bigger on the left side than on the right, and this is true even in newborn babies. Could this kind of anatomical asymmetry be the material expression of Chomsky's innate capacity for human language? If so, then it is difficult to explain why a young child can apparently develop the speech mechanisms in his right hemisphere if the left side is damaged; and even harder to explain the fact that gorillas and chimpanzees have the same anatomical asymmetry, though Chomsky would deny them the capacity for language.

There is no denying, of course, that speech *seems* to outstrip in complexity any animal communication system that we understand. But I wonder if we are not missing immense subtlety in the behaviour of animals. Indeed, it is inconceivable, as Chomsky points out, that monkeys and apes have the *capacity* for language but

144

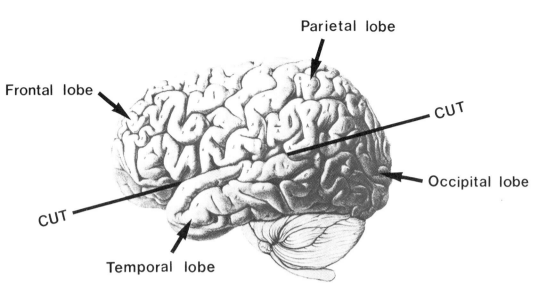

Frontal lobe

Parietal lobe

CUT

Occipital lobe

CUT

Temporal lobe

Wernicke's area is larger on the left side in the majority of humans. N. Geschwind and W. Levitsky examined a large number of human brains cut along the Sylvian fissure, which divides the temporal lobe from the parietal lobe. The diagram below is a view from above after the top of the brain has been lifted off, revealing the upper surface of the temporal lobes. The shaded region, called the temporal plane, *is part of Wernicke's area and is bigger on the left side. This region may be involved in the analysis of speech; damage to Wernicke's area often leads to an inability to understand speech correctly although the patient is still able to talk, albeit not perfectly. On the right side of the brain, the region behind the temporal plane, part of the parietal lobe, is correspondingly larger; the right parietal lobe seems to be specialized for complex visual functions, such as perception of distance and spatial relationships. This anatomical asymmetry is present as early as the thirty-first week of human fetal life, and also exists in the chimpanzee's brain.*

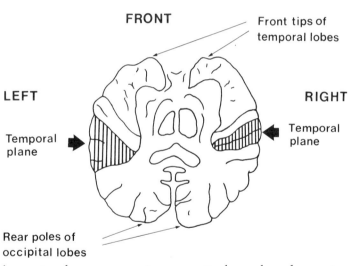

FRONT

Front tips of temporal lobes

LEFT

RIGHT

Temporal plane

Temporal plane

Rear poles of occipital lobes

have simply never put it to use. Perhaps they do use it, but we cannot comprehend them. Take, for instance, this description of an encounter between two male *lemurs*, usually considered relatively primitive primates:

'The *lemur* stares towards another animal. He draws his upper lip forward and down, so that it covers the points of his canines and protrudes somewhat below the lower jaw . . . but the lips are tense and do not droop. The ex-

145

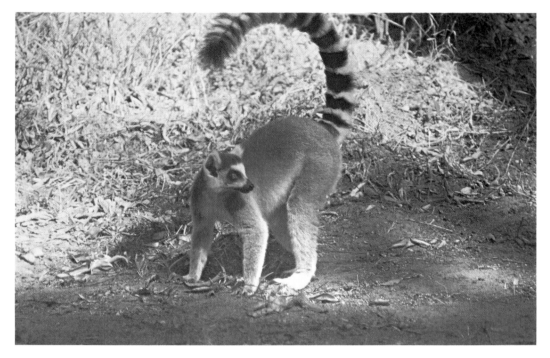

The tail-waving stink fight of a male ring-tailed lemur, described by Alison Jolley and photographed by Hugh Fraser Rowell.

pression probably flares the nostrils. He may either squeal or purr. He then stands on all fours with his tail arched over his back, its tip just above his head. He quivers the tail violently . . . shaking its odor forward.'

Are we any better equipped to interpret the syntax of this message than the lemur is to decipher our speech? Even the most ceremonial communication by animals *appears* to us to be stereotyped and thus lacking in rich information content, but we may be unable to comprehend the variety of signals available through the *combination* of different modes of expression.

But *speech*, as the vehicle of true language, *is* unique to man, and its special quality, which makes it so very powerful, is that the single medium can be used for the combination of signals which animals might transmit in different modalities (movement, smell, touch and vocalization). How could speaking itself possibly have evolved?

The answer might lie, like the key to so much of man's

development, in his bipedal posture and the increasing skill and sensitivity of his hands, freed from the drudgery of weight-bearing or swinging through the trees. The precision grip of man's hands matured over the period between five million and two and a half million years ago, and during that time his brain doubled in size, perhaps to accommodate the increasingly sophisticated mechanisms for planning and controlling individual movements of the fingers and, even more, the skilled *sequences* of hand and body movement needed for inventiveness in the manipulation of objects. The earliest stone tools yet discovered date from the end of this period, and so, I suspect, does the flowering of language, though not speech. Perhaps man suddenly found that his newly-nimble fingers and the computational power of his brain allowed him to expand and enrich one aspect of the communication of his primate ancestors, the very one that Washoe and Lucy have learned to exploit – gesture. The blossoming of communication in early man might have involved a florid system of gestural signalling with hands and face, even including music-making and dance.

Now one disadvantage of communication by gesture is that it demands constant visual attention from the

This is a spectrogram – a record of the tones and their intensities in human speech. The dimensions of the display are the frequency of sound (on the vertical axis), time (on the horizontal axis) and the intensity of sound (represented by the darkness of the trace). This particular spectrogram, prepared by Mark Haggard, shows the words /ku/('coo') and /ki/('key') uttered by a man. Each word consists of the /k/ consonant at the beginning with the vowel sound following it. Each vowel is a relatively static and different set of frequency bands, called formants, represented by the horizontal striations, but the burst portion of the /k/ sound, indicated by the arrow above each word, is totally different in its frequency components in these two examples, even though it is heard as the same consonant. In 'coo', the /k/ is softer, shorter and much lower in frequency than it is in 'key'. However, in 'coo' the dominant formant of the 'oo' vowel is the second formant, about 1 kilohertz in frequency: in the 'ee' vowel of 'key' the third formant, about 3 kilohertz, is dominant. So in each case the burst of the /k/ consists mainly of frequencies similar to, or just above, the dominant formant of the following vowel; the place of articulation of the consonant is said to be assimilated to that of the vowel. The listener must take the total acoustical form into account in order to perceive the spoken word. Infants take longer to learn to understand and speak consonants like /k/, which vary in sound content, than other less variable consonants.

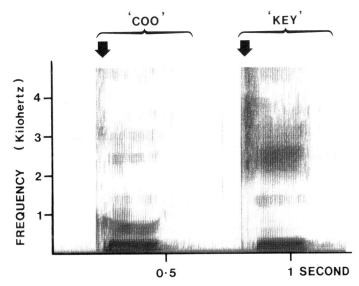

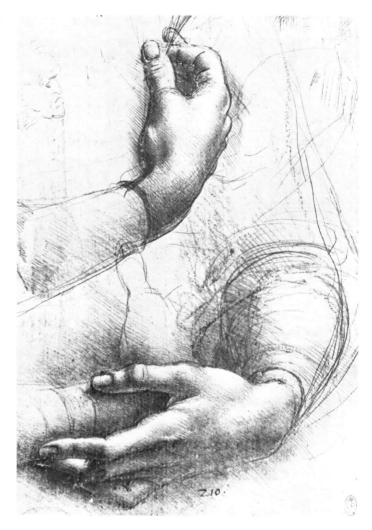

The precision grip of man's hands.
Studies by Leonardo da Vinci.

receiver of the signal. There would have been considerable benefit if one of the hands had become specialized for transmitting messages, so that anyone watching for a signal could reliably predict from what direction it would come. This might have been the reason for the appearance of general left cerebral dominance, and hence right-handedness. The emergence of common handedness would then have brought many secondary advantages, for instance in the sharing of tools, in coordinating skilled communal labour and in social exchanges, dances and ceremonies.

148

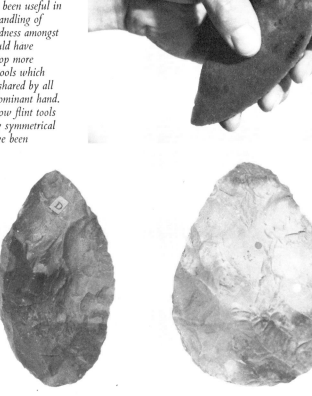

Dominant right-handedness may have evolved in early man as an aid in gestural communication. The emergence of heightened skill in one hand would also have been useful in the construction and handling of tools. Common handedness amongst a group of people would have allowed them to develop more complicated 'handed' tools which could then have been shared by all those with the same dominant hand. These photographs show flint tools that are not bilaterally symmetrical and therefore may have been

constructed and used by men with dominant hands. The upper tool is perhaps an implement for scraping (approximately 50,000 years old, probably made by Neanderthal man). The curved, sharp edge was almost certainly made by holding the stone, as shown, in the left hand and turning it back and forth by bending the wrist, while carefully chipping away the edge with a hammer held in the skilled right hand. The curvature of the edge is centred on the rotating point of the left wrist.

The lower tools are hand axes (probably made by Homo erectus, *about 100,000 years ago). They have been made with a twist in them, perhaps to facilitate their being held in the right hand. Hand axes twisted in the opposite direction have also been found, but are less common.*

Two experimental observations bear on this theory of the gestural origin of human communication. First, just as the growth of a human embryo seems to be a cryptic summary of man's biological evolution, so the development of language in the human infant may include the cultural predecessor of speech. For very young babies, before they can speak, seem to communicate mainly through gesticulation and expressive movements of the face. The second line of evidence comes from a clinical procedure for testing cerebral dominance before neuro-surgical operations. A short-lasting anaesthetic is injected into one of the two carotid arteries which supply blood separately to the two cerebral hemispheres. This puts one hemisphere out of action for a short time and the patient's speech is tested to discover whether its mecha-

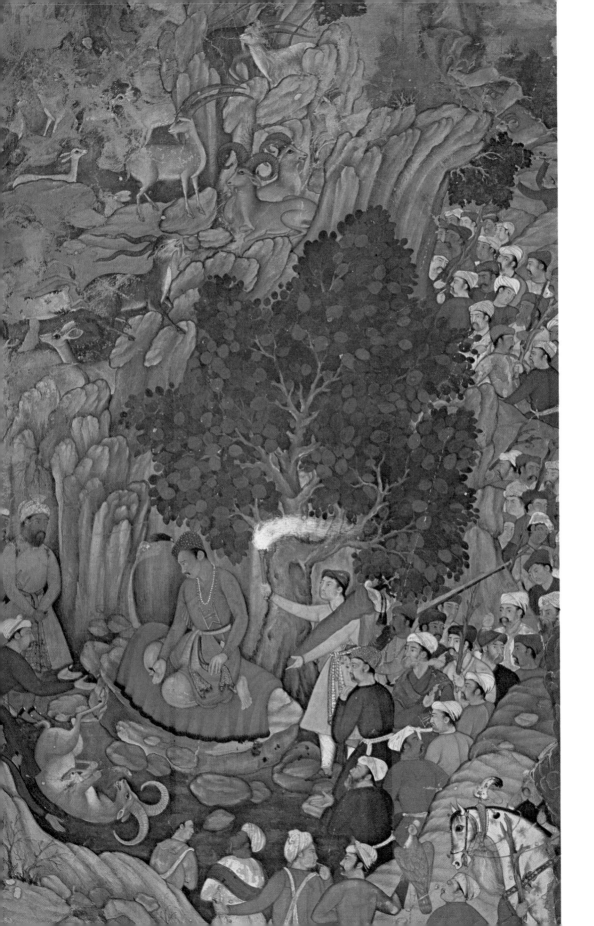

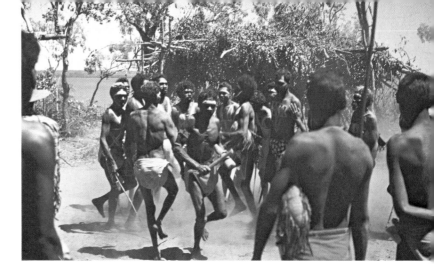

Gunavidji aborigines of Maningrida, north-eastern Australia, perform a ritual ceremony to invoke ancestral spirits. The aborigines may have a life-style similar to that of early man. They use a silent gestural language, especially during hunting. Photograph by David Attenborough.

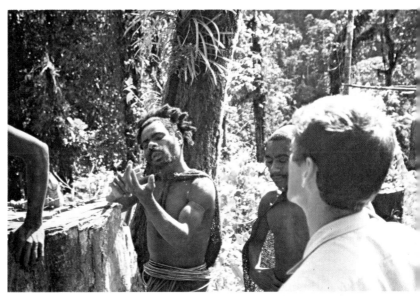

The Biami people of central New Guinea, employ a gestural system for counting. They use their fingers to count from one to ten and then continue with wrist, elbow, upper arm, shoulder and neck to reach fifteen. There are probably about 1000 spoken languages in New Guinea, but distinctive gestural systems of counting are much smaller in number. They have been used by anthropologists to establish cultural relationships between groups with different spoken languages. Photograph by David Attenborough.

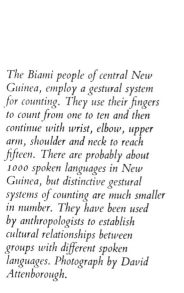

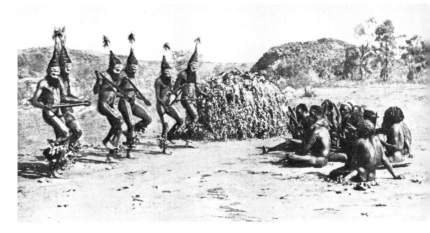

B. Spencer and F. J. Gillen, in the 1920s, studied the gestural language of the Arunta aborigines, as well as their ceremonies. This is one of Spencer and Gillen's photographs, showing a dance in the Tjitjingalla Corroboree.

151

The emperor Akbar converted from hunting. Moghul miniature, c. 1590, from Abul Fazl's Akbarnama.

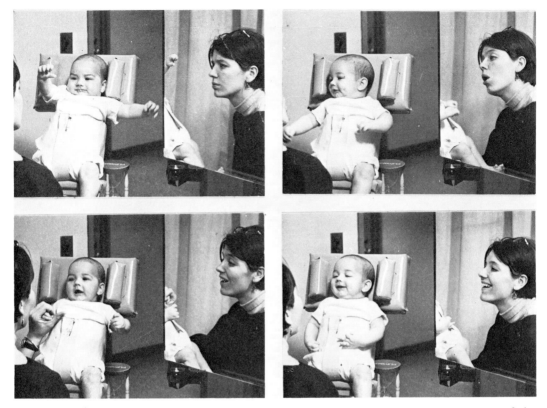

Colwyn Trevarthen has studied the 'dialogue' between infant and mother. He believes that it consists of gesticulation and 'prespeech' – almost voiceless movements of lips and tongue – on the part of the baby, and exaggerated mimickry of the baby by its mother. The mother's face is reflected in a mirror, allowing the photographer to capture her responses as well as the baby's.

nism is localized on that side of the brain. Now if the patient is taught a series of hand gestures before the injection, he cannot perform them when the speech hemisphere is anaesthetized. The programming of skilled gesticulations and speech share the same side of the brain.

The explosive development of speech itself may have happened only 100,000 years or less before the present time (a mere moment ago in evolutionary terms). The gradual transition from a meat-hunting and plant-gathering life-style to a society based on agriculture must have put increasing emphasis on the ability to make long-term plans and to consult past experiences. No doubt man had always added his inherited stock of primate vocalizations to his gestural conversations to give them emotional force; the bold new step was to exploit this repertoire of sounds and to bestow on it the grammatical power that had already been developed, first for the construction of tools and then for gestural communication.

There are several legendary tales of the search for the origin of man's language. Psammethicus, a Pharoah of Egypt, is said to have had two newborn infants reared by a silent shepherd who fed them with goat's milk. According to the tale, they taught themselves to say the word 'becos', which Psammethicus discovered was the Phrygian word for 'bread'. James IV of Scotland is supposed to have done a similar experiment, and his pair of 'bairnes' came out speaking 'guid Hebrew'.

But the most convincing story of all is of the Moghul emperor Akbar Khan, who interned twelve babies with dumb nurses in a castle six leagues from Akbar's capital of Agra. 'When the children were twelve years old,' wrote the Jesuit Father Catrou in 1705, 'he had them brought before him, and collected in his palace men skilled in all languages . . . When however the children appeared before the Emperor, everyone was astonished to find that they did not *speak* any language at all. They had learnt from their nurses to do without any, and they merely expressed their thoughts by *gestures* which answered the purpose of words.' Perhaps Akbar's twelve infants *had* discovered the true origin of human language.

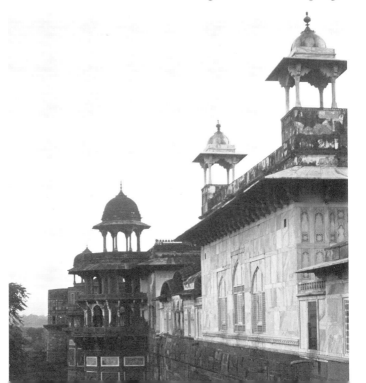

Akbar's Palace, the Red Fort at Agra.

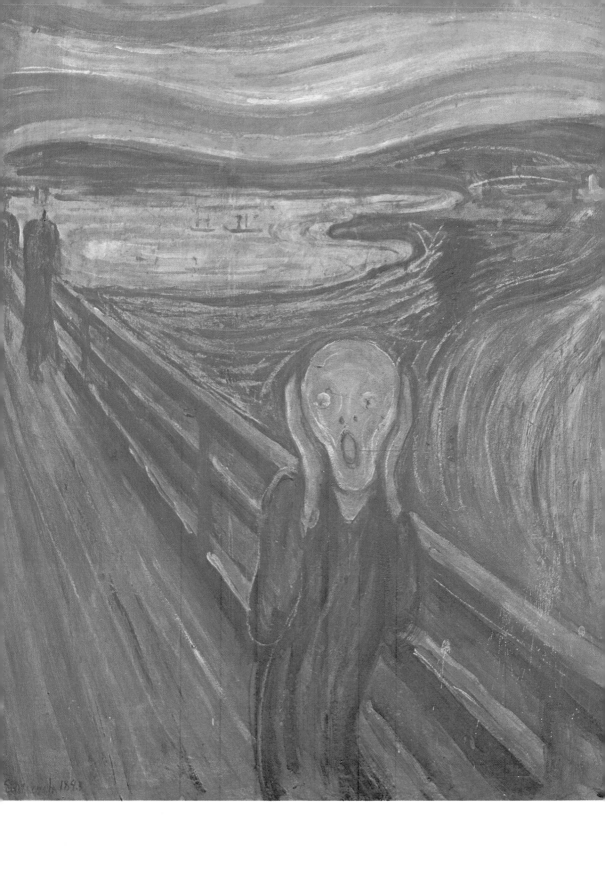

6

Madness and morality

I was walking along the road with two friends.
The sun set. I felt a tinge of melancholy.
Suddenly the sky became a bloody red.

I stopped and leaned against the railing, dead
tired, and looked at the flaming clouds that
hung like blood and a sword over the blue-black
fjord and the city.

My friends walked on. I stood there, trembling
with fright. And I felt a loud, unending scream
piercing nature.

Edvard Munch (1863–1944)

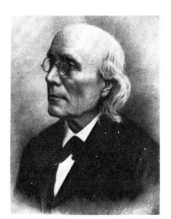

Gustav Theodor Fechner
(1801–1887).

◀

'The Scream', 1893, by Edvard
Munch (1863–1944).

Gustav Fechner was the founder of a new and objective approach to the measurement of mental events, a concept that he crystallized in the name that he coined for his science – psychophysics. Fechner hoped that the kind of strict experiments that had beaten the forces of Nature into the laws of physics could work for the mind of man as well. Yet despite the orderly, reductionist nature of his ideas, Fechner, in 1860, permitted himself an extraordinary speculation about personal consciousness. The brain, he knew, is bilaterally symmetrical; it has two sides, which are virtually mirror-images of each other. Nowhere is this clearer than in the cerebral hemispheres; there is a deep cleft between the two halves, which are linked by an enormous strap, containing millions of nerve fibres – the *corpus callosum*. If consciousness is a property of the brain (which Fechner certainly believed),

155

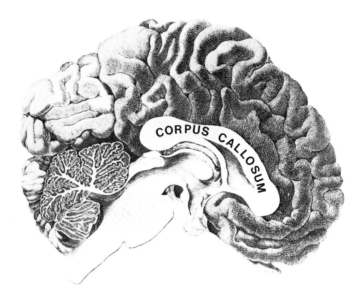

CORPUS CALLOSUM

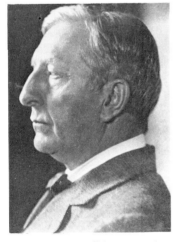

Soemmerring's (1796) diagram of the human brain sectioned down the middle shows the corpus callosum very clearly.

William McDougall (1871–1938).

what would happen if the cerebral hemispheres were literally split apart completely? As the psychologist William McDougall reported in 1911, Fechner asserted 'that if a man's brain could be mechanically divided into two parts (as by the transection of the *corpus callosum*) without arresting the life of the parts, the nervous activities of each part would be accompanied by its own stream of consciousness'. In other words, Fechner believed that one mind would become two if the brain that kept it caged were cut in half. McDougall himself, however, was convinced that no mere split in the brain could divide the mind.

Fechner, of course, thought that this experiment would never and could never be done. And McDougall surely believed the same, though he taunted the eminent Oxford physiologist Sir Charles Sherrington with a request that if he, McDougall, were ever struck by an incurable disease, Sherrington himself should operate on him and cut his *corpus callosum*. 'If I am right,' he said, 'my consciousness will remain a unitary consciousness.'

The hypothetical, inconceivable experiment of Fechner and McDougall has actually been performed; and its results are, quite simply, some of the most fascinating

156

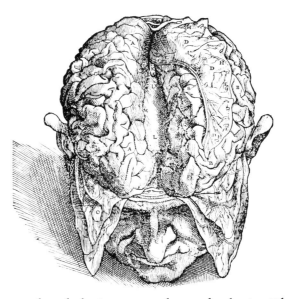

This illustration from De Fabrica *(1543) by Andreas Vesalius shows the corpus callosum (L) connecting together the two cerebral hemispheres.*

produced during research on the brain. The rationale behind this unlikely story is that an epileptic seizure originating at a focus of damage on one side of the brain can spread to the other hemisphere through the nerve fibres of the *corpus callosum*. The attack then takes on the terrible proportions of a *grand mal* convulsion, involving the whole body. Nowadays the treatment of epilepsy with palliative drugs is quite successful, but in a few cases the fits become worse and worse, until the regular occurrence of seizures, sometimes many each day, makes normal life impossible. Now in California, in the 1950s, experiments with animals had demonstrated that cutting the *corpus callosum* did not interfere in a gross way with movement or any vital function. So a bold (some would say reckless) surgeon decided to split the *corpus callosum* in a few patients who had intractable epilepsy, hoping that it would moderate their fits. It did – to an unexpected extent. Not only did the convulsions no longer involve both sides of the body, but they were reduced in frequency too, though the reason for this therapeutic bonus is still unknown. But what of the other consequences of this unlikely invasion of the mind; who was right, Fechner or McDougall?

157

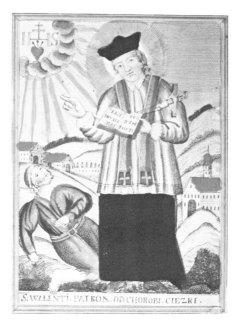

St Valentin, patron saint of epileptics.

S. WALENTI. PATRON. OD CHOROBI. CIEZKI.

LAQVINTACOIA
CHINBOMAMA
CAVA

Felipe Guaman Poma de Ayala, c. 1613, depicted with accuracy the mal de corason *or epileptic fits, suffered by the fifth Inca Queen Chimbomamacava.*
From Nueva coronica y Buen Gobierno.

Reyno hasta quichiua aymara

chinbo

Roger Sperry and his collaborators, at the California Institute of Technology, who had already done much of the preliminary work with animals, had the chance to examine these people whose brains had been split. At first, apart from the usual after-effects of any neurosurgical operation, the patients seemed remarkably normal; indeed that had always been the conclusion in previous studies of people who had suffered damage to the *corpus callosum*. However, careful and often ingenious testing revealed a bizarre mental syndrome. It is surely significant that Sperry made one of the first reports of his studies at a conference entitled 'Brain and Conscious Experience', at the Pontifical Academy of Sciences – a meeting that was addressed by Pope Paul VI. In Sperry's own words, in his report to that conference: 'Everything we have seen so far indicates that the surgery has left these people with two separate minds, that is two separate spheres of consciousness. What is experienced in the right hemisphere seems to be entirely outside the realm of awareness of the left.'

Roger Sperry took advantage of the fact that the connections to and from one hemisphere are principally concerned with the opposite side of the body. If a split-brain patient is blindfolded, and some familiar object, like a comb or a coin, is put into one hand, he can use that same hand to retrieve the object from a collection of similar things by touch alone. But ask the other hand to do it and the result is pure guesswork. Imagine the patient looking fixedly at a point when a picture of an object is flashed momentarily just to the left of that point (so that it is seen only by the right hemisphere, because of the distribution of nerve fibres from the eyes to the brain). Now, the patient can select the object portrayed by sight, or even by touch alone, when he uses his left hand, but not his right, to choose from an array of objects.

Each hemisphere, then, seems whole in itself, but with

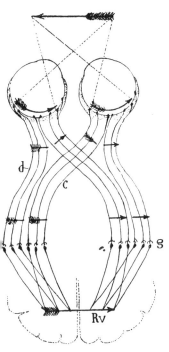

Santiago Ramón y Cajal's diagram (1899) of the projection of nerves from the eyes to the brain shows how, in both eyes, the left-hand half of the retina (which receives images from the right side of visual space) sends its fibres to the left side of the brain. Each hemisphere, then, has access to visual information from the opposite half of the visual field.

159

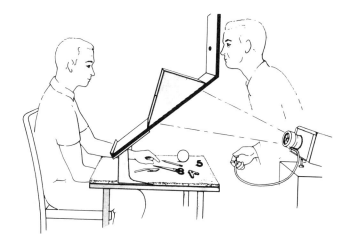

only half a body to serve it. Judged by any simple criterion, like seeing, feeling, remembering or moving, there is not much to choose between the skills of the two hemispheres. To that extent Fechner was correct. Indeed, Sperry's descriptions convey an eerie impression that the split-brain patient is no longer one person, but two; both hands do indeed have minds of their own.

But 'mind-left' and 'mind-right' are not equal in every respect. The biggest difference between them (or at least the most immediate) is that one hemisphere – the left in all of Sperry's patients – does the talking. Put an object in the right hand or flash a picture on the right of the visual field, and the patient, or rather his left hemisphere, can tell you what it is. But show it on the left side, so that only the right hemisphere knows about it, and the articulate left is lost for words. So the mind that makes its presence felt, because it can speak, is that of the so-called major hemisphere, usually the left. To that extent, McDougall was correct. The speechlessness of the right hemisphere has been seized upon by some as evidence that the consciousness of man cannot be truly divided. But such an argument seems to me quite specious – rather like saying that a brain-damaged patient who simply cannot speak, but understands speech perfectly well, is not conscious and is therefore not human.

160

The minor, right hemisphere is not even totally illiterate; it can read. When the word 'comb' is flashed on the left of a screen, so that only the right hemisphere can see it, the patient cannot *say* what was written but can reach with his left hand and select the correct object from a choice. If a picture of a steaming cup of coffee is shown to the right hemisphere, the left hand can point out, amongst an array of cards, the one with the word 'hot' written on it. So adjectives as well as nouns are understood by 'mind-right'. But all the time the left hemisphere, speaking through the mouth of the patient, has no idea what is going on. By all accounts the right hemisphere is not very good with verbs, but it does have the vocabulary and the syntactical ability of a young child.

And what is more, in certain respects the subordinate right *excels* over the 'dominant' left. It is much *better* at any job that involves recognizing patterns and shapes, and particularly complicated solid objects. The right hemisphere can draw quite well with its left hand but the left hemisphere even has problems in copying simple

A split-brain patient was asked to draw or write answers to spoken questions and commands. The verbal signals, spoken by the experimenter, are listed on the left, and the responses of the right hand and left hand are shown next to them. Both hemispheres seemed to understand the spoken words but only the left hemisphere (right hand) was able to write its reply. The right hemisphere (left hand) could, however, draw simple geometrical shapes on spoken command. These results were collected six months after the operation. By a couple of months later, the patient had become quite good at writing with her left hand, but probably not because the right hemisphere had learned how to do so; almost certainly the left hemisphere had learned to control the left hand through the very small fraction of motor nerve fibres from the brain to the hands that do not cross over to the opposite side. (Adapted from Fig. 13 of Gazzaniga, 1970.)

	R. HAND	L. HAND
"This is a pretty day"	*This is a pretty day*	
"Your name"	*Nancy*	
"Square"		
"Circle"		
"Triangle"		

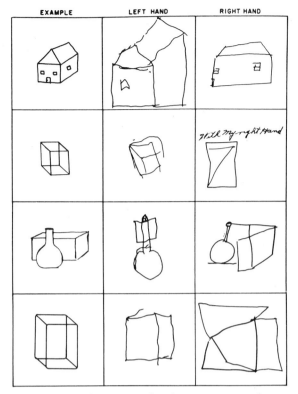

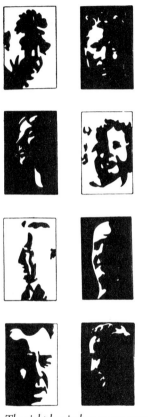

The right hemisphere seems generally superior to the left in any task that involves complex visual recognition. These silhouette drawings, designed by Craig Mooney, test the ability to construct a whole, meaningful percept out of fragmentary information. Patients whose right hemispheres have been injured often have great difficulty in perceiving the faces in these drawings.

diagrams of houses and cubes – it is much more at home writing than drawing. Recognizing faces, surely an immensely important part of human social behaviour, is also apparently a speciality of the so-called 'minor' hemisphere.

Fascinating though these observations on split-brain people are, I believe that they have been misinterpreted in their relevance to the functions of the normal human brain. Protagonists of different factions have all nurtured the idea that you and I have virtually independent sides to our brains and therefore to our intellects. The dominant side, usually the left, talks, writes, does mathematics, and thinks in a logical, serial way; the minor right side recognizes shapes and faces, appreciates music, puts on its owner's clothes, and works in a global, intuitive fashion. The verbal ordered culture of the Western world, dominated by scientific and technological progress, is, we are told, managed by the left hemispheres

162

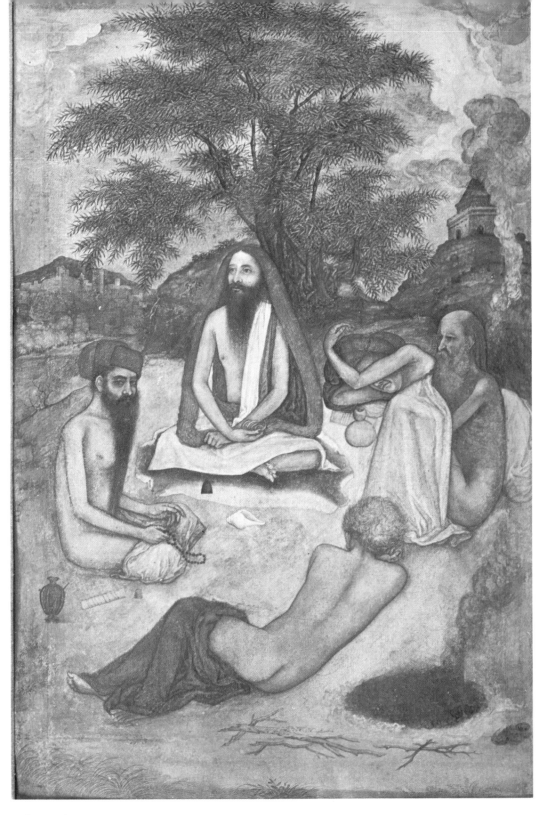

*Gathering of yogis, discussing with
their left hemispheres the thoughts
of their right. Moghul miniature
painting by Govardhan, 1620.*

of its populations; the mystical, artistic and religious cultures of the East must be driven by their right hemispheres.

There is a growing, vocal movement that calls (presumably with its left hemisphere) for the liberation of its right. Some psychologists, most vociferously Robert Ornstein, want a revolution in Western education with more emphasis on non-verbal skills and the special attributes of the minor hemisphere, which are supposed to rule the cultures of the East. One cannot help feeling that some Oriental Robert Ornstein, contemplating the material progress that those attributes of the left hemisphere have given to the Western world, might make just the opposite recommendation.

In fact, Hugh Sykes Davies, the scholar of English, recently attacked the 'rightist' movement, and complained that verbal skills are degenerating, not dominating, in our society. All this fiery rhetoric seems to me to be based on a curious assumption that the two hemispheres of a normal man are as divided as those of Sperry's patients. Under exceptional circumstances, in unusual people, the separate characteristics of the two halves of the brain might come into conflict. The author

Recent experiments on split-brain patients have revealed the superiority of the right hemisphere in recognizing faces. As in the earlier tests, the patient looks fixedly at a spot on a screen, but instead of the experimenter flashing a picture or word to only one side of the screen or the other (so that only one hemisphere sees it), in the recent tests, a 'split-picture' is projected in such a way that one half of the picture falls to the right, the other half to the left of the fixation point. Now, when such a picture is briefly exposed (so that the eyes have insufficient time to shift their gaze) both hemispheres see a different pattern at the same time. In the example shown above, the picture used is a split-face, made up of two half faces. If the patient is asked to say what he has seen, he (his left hemisphere) will describe the face that fell to the right of the fixation point; but if asked to choose from a set of photographs by pointing, he almost invariably picks the face that his right hemisphere saw, even if he uses his right hand, which is only under partial control of the right hemisphere.

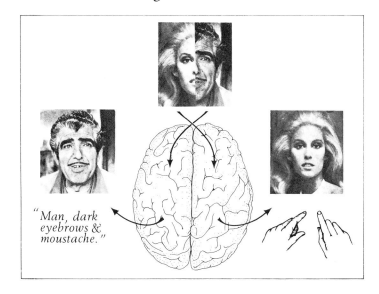

"Man, dark eyebrows & moustache."

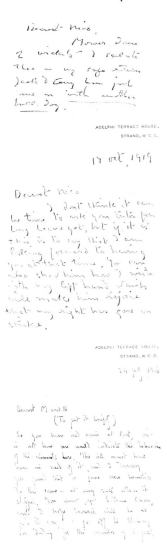

Three examples of J. M. Barrie's handwriting. The first is a letter, written in 1918, with his right hand. Barrie was naturally left-handed but had been forced at school to use his right. The second letter (1919) was one of the first that he wrote with his left hand. The final example (1926) shows his later left-handed style.

J. M. Barrie, for instance, was ambidextrous; he even wrote his plays with either hand, and his desk is worn smooth on both sides to prove it. He was sure that his two hands had different characters and that he was inhabited by two different people. But in most of us there is a constant traffic of information between the two hemispheres, a tying-together of separate experiences, a sharing of special talents.

Even in split-brain people, the ability of the two sides of the brain to whisper to each other in the subtlest of ways is quite remarkable. Take the case of one experiment in which a spot of light, either red or green, was flashed to the right hemisphere and the split-brain patient was asked to say what colour he had seen. Both hemispheres understood the question but, of course, only the left could reply, so it simply guessed the answer, and therefore got it wrong half the time. But to Sperry's surprise, if allowed a second chance to correct himself, the patient always got the answer right. What seemed to be happening was this: the mute right hemisphere heard the guess of its verbose leftist colleague and if the answer was wrong, the right hemisphere triggered an intense emotional reaction. The patient frowned, blushed and shook his head immediately after making the faulty guess; and the left hemisphere, detecting the dissatisfaction of the knowledgeable right, quickly changed its mind and corrected itself. If the cerebral hemispheres are capable of this kind of collaboration with no overt connections at all between them, how much more certain should they be to share their skills when they have millions of fibres in the *corpus callosum* to bind them together!

What we should be striving to achieve for ourselves and our brains is not the pampering of one hemisphere to the neglect of the other (whether right or left), or their independent development, but the marriage and harmony of the two. It so happens that the special mental

Theories of how animals learn generally involve the idea that some kind of 'rewarding' or 'reinforcing' signal must arrive in the brain in order to increase the probability that an animal will repeat its previously successful actions. The reinforcing signal is presumably the sensory activity set up by eating, drinking, sex and so on. Experiments, started by James Olds and Peter Milner in the early fifties, pointed to various parts of the brain stem as reward centres or 'pleasure centres', which might be involved in the reception of reinforcing messages. They discovered that if an electrode is permanently and painlessly implanted at any one of a vast number of points in a rat's brain, and it is connected up in such a manner that the rat can deliver a shock to the electrode by pressing a lever, the animal will do so, time after time, even to the total neglect of genuine bodily requirements, as if the normal actions associated with learning had been by-passed and the electrode had found the site of pure reinforcement. Here, in an experiment by Tim Crow and Gordon Arbuthnott, a rat is 'self-stimulating'. The present evidence suggests that parts of the brain-stem where neurons use the substances noradrenaline and dopamine as their transmitter substances (described in chapters 2 and 3), may be the sites of reinforcement. There were hopes (or fears) that implantation of electrodes into the 'pleasure centres' of the human brain might become commonplace as treatment for the depressed or as titillation for the hedonistic. Fortunately it seems that the sensations produced by such stimulation in man are rarely intensely pleasurable, though the technique has been used on some patients in states of intense and incurable pain.

A view of the future, or an unfounded fear? An illustration from the magazine Psychology Today.

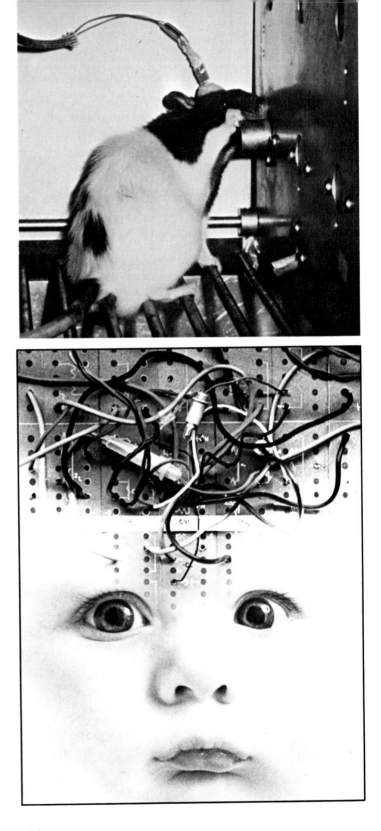

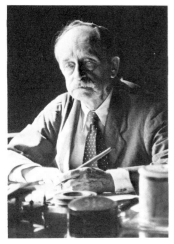

J. M. Barrie at his desk.

Left hemisphere consults right? George Harrison joins in a chant with the London branch of the International Society for Krishna Consciousness.

territories of the minor, right hemisphere – spatial perception, pictorial recognition and intuitive thought – are not easily amenable to conventional education, nor is it clear that they would benefit from years of formal instruction. Systems of education, especially higher education (and this applies to every culture) seem designed to develop and exploit the powers of the hemisphere that is dominant for speech, for those powers depend most on factual knowledge and prolonged training.

The ripening of cerebral dominance is one of the most important processes in the maturation of the brain. Unitary control of delicate motor skills, like speech and the fine movements of the dominant hand, requires the firm planting of the special apparatus for their control in one side of the brain. To ignore the special role and the particular educational needs of the dominant hemisphere, and to encourage the minor side to take charge may produce deleterious consequences in behaviour. It could cause problems as profound as the disorders of emotion and speech, especially stuttering, that are attributed to

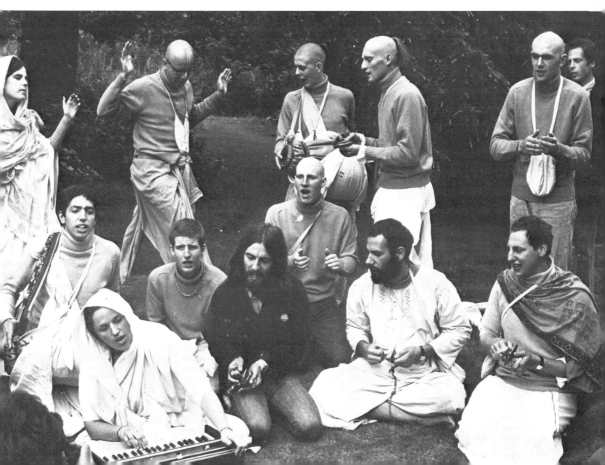

another cultural interference with cerebral dominance – the forced use of the right hand in naturally left-handed children. This form of social brain control was common in Europe and the United States, and was virtually mandatory in the Soviet Union, until quite recently.

The debate about liberating the minor hemisphere is only a fashionable twist to an ancient and inextinguishable aspiration of man – to control his brain; or, more often, to control someone else's. The brain is the organ of behaviour, and the dream of every leader, whether a tyrannical despot or a benign prophet, is to regulate the behaviour of his people. There is a growing fear that a considerable fraction of brain research is aimed at making such control a reality.

It is true that animals will work ceaselessly to receive electrical stimulation through electrodes implanted in so-called 'pleasure centres' in their brains. The most effective areas lie in the hypothalamus (which is involved in the regulation of motivated behaviour, like eating, drinking and sex) and in the nearby limbic system (which is thought to control emotions like rage, fear and joy). It is also true that electrical stimulation at certain sites or local damage at others can calm the fiercest beast or turn a placid animal into a savage killer. The physiologist J. F. Fulton wrote that a certain tiny injury to a monkey's brain 'yields an animal that is formidably ferocious ... I finally had to decree that no one should ever examine [such a] monkey alone, for ... they attack to kill, and they single out the examiner's neck as their initial objective. The aggressive behaviour comes in waves and is accompanied by salivation ... baring of the teeth, and a kind of guttural vocalization that one seldom hears in a normal monkey.'

There is, naturally, widespread apprehension, nurtured by popular publications and not always discouraged by over-enthusiastic experimenters, that such techniques will soon be part and parcel of everyday life.

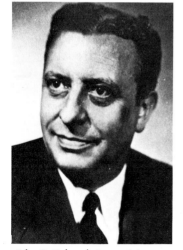

John F. Fulton (1899–1960).

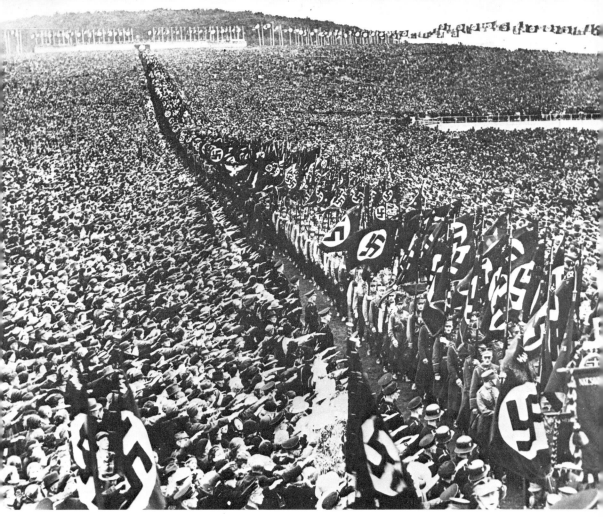

Implanted electrodes are not needed for control of behaviour. Nazi rally in pre-war Germany.

Such fears are, in the main, quite unfounded; fortunately, the sheer paraphernalia of experimental brain manipulation, the implanted electrodes, the cables and electronics, the tedious surgical techniques, make that kind of brain control beyond the reach of any modern-day Alexander or Genghis Khan who wishes to motivate an army or subjugate the world at the push of a button. And in any case, are our brains not already more totally disciplined, our opinions more firmly moulded, and our minds more sharply directed by the political and social environment, than by any electrode that could be put in our heads? The stentorian voices of the mass media are more universally powerful than the indiscriminate persuasions of any mind-altering drug.

169

More illuminating than pointing an accusing finger at the motives of brain research is to ask *why* society always has attempted to regulate and order the behaviour of its members. The answer might lie in a very basic biological need to identify – in order to identify *with*.

Kin selection is a term used to describe the operation of evolutionary forces on closely-knit and inter-breeding groups of animals, not just individuals; it was recognized by Charles Darwin as an important factor in the emergence of social behaviour. By forming collaborative groups, largely based on family ties, animals can improve their chances of surviving as a group, and hence of propagating their common genes. Biologists even seek to explain the most cherished of human ethical principles – altruism, heroism and unselfishness – in terms of kin selection of shared genetic material. J. B. S. Haldane once remarked that he was willing to lay down his life – for two brothers or eight cousins!

Now the preservation of common genes amongst a social group, by such acts of cooperation and self-

Is discrimination today a cultural exaggeration of the logic of kin selection? A segregated bridge in Cape Town, South Africa.

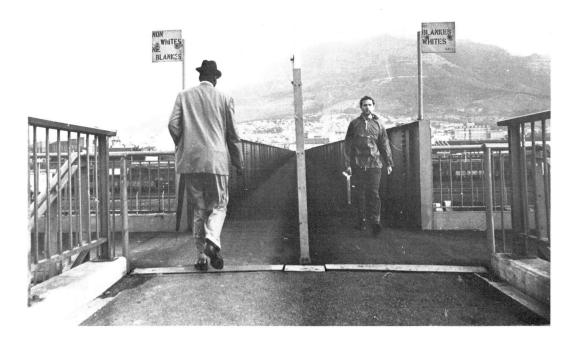

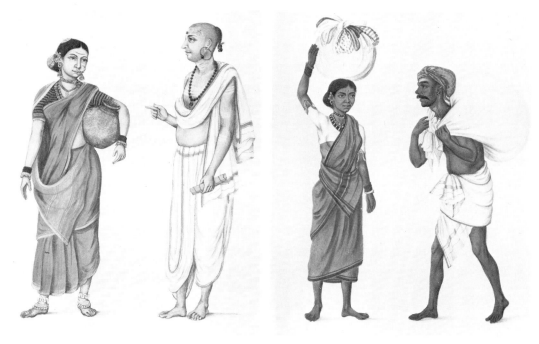

The caste structure of India. Left, Shaiva Brahmin and wife. Right, Dhobi (washerman) and wife. Water-colour drawings, c. 1828, made by Indian artists for the guidance of Europeans in India

sacrifice, would be greatly enhanced by an ability of the individual to recognize in others those similarities in appearance and behaviour that betray shared genes. One of the major factors in the evolution of human society is the specialization of the brain to recognize and classify. That power, which has all sorts of cultural ramifications, in perception, language and even aesthetics, may have had its origin in the discrimination of genetic similarities and dissimilarities in other men. An animal, like man, that could actively direct its altruism and shape its behavioural ethics to protect its own genetically similar colleagues would have had an enormous advantage in kin selection. The roots of social discrimination today, then, lie in the group discrimination of yesterday. The intolerance of difference has produced such social cancers as apartheid in South Africa, the caste structure of India and the endless warfare of Europe. Consider too the scientific argument about genetic inheritance of intelligence, which rages back and forth; do blacks in the United States have slightly lower average

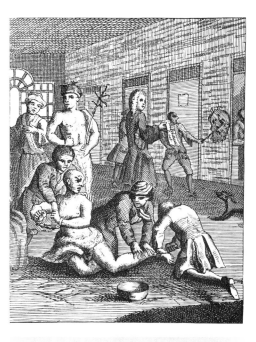

A ward in Bethlem Hospital, c. 1745. Bethlem Royal Hospital (Bedlam) was designed by the physicist Robert Hooke and was built in 1675–6 as part of the reconstruction of London after the Great Fire. Bethlem Hospital was originally founded as a priory in Bishopsgate, London, in 1247, and was the oldest public asylum in Europe, except for that at Granada in Spain.

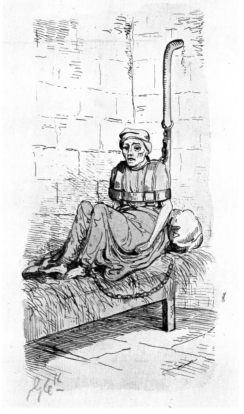

William Norris (died 1815) was an American who was confined in Bethlem Hospital for twelve years, bound by chains, one foot long, to an iron rod at the head of his bed. Etching (1815) by George Cruikshank from a drawing by G. Arnald, which was exhibited to a Select Committee on Madhouses set up by the House of Commons in 1815.

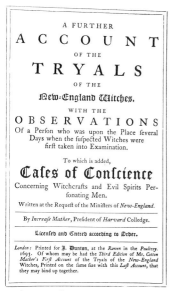

Title page of an eye-witness account of the trial of witches at Salem, Massachusetts, in 1692. Twenty people were executed in one year. Many of the victims of the 'witchcraft' were young girls who had violent fits and spasms of choking, and complained of being pinched, pricked and bitten by 'specters', which they saw as dreadful hallucinations. A very recent theory, proposed by Linnda Caporael, suggests that the symptoms described may not have been those of 'witchcraft', but of poisoning by ergot, a fungus that can infect rye, used to make bread. Ergot is chemically related to LSD, which probably acts by interfering with chemical transmission at synapses in the brain. Ergot poisoning does seem to affect women and children more than men; it can cause muscular spasm (and hence choking), crawling and pricking sensations and visual hallucinations.

St Zenobius casting out a devil. Panel from an altarpiece by Pesellino (c. 1422–1457), The National Gallery, London.

scores than whites on conventional tests of intelligence because of genetic or environmental factors? The motive behind the question is the identification of difference – as if such differences could *justify* racial discrimination.

Many of the most precious elements in human social behaviour, such as formalized sexual bonding and family structure, rich communal ceremony and the embracing of ethical principles within religious codes, can be viewed as deliberate cultural exaggerations of inherited components of behaviour that favour kin selection. The desire to regulate behaviour, even to bring deviants back to the norm, may be a further cultural embellishment of the logic of kin selection.

Nowhere is this more evident than in the field of mental disease, where the questions of social intolerance of difference and the danger of active brain control become most profound. The problem of illness of the mind is a challenge not only to medicine but also to society. Each year one man in fourteen, one woman in seven, consults a doctor about some form of mental disease; every year 600,000 people in Great Britain are referred to psychiatrists. Because the very symptoms of mental disease are defined as aberrations of behaviour, they bring the sufferer into conflict with the community,

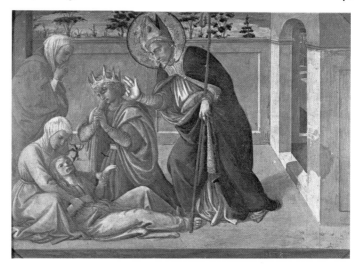

173

in a way that no illness of any other organ can. Diseases of the mind are an insult to the behavioural order on which society rests. Most of all, they are usually disorders of emotion, a function that the human mind has so carefully concealed under its cognitive skin.

It is no coincidence that, in history, the same treatments have been meted out to the mentally sick as to those other offenders against the order of society – the criminal and the heretic. At best they have had their demons cast out or merely been imprisoned; at worst they have been tortured to death. Textbooks of psychiatry try to achieve the same as the codes of secular law or religious commandments; they all attempt to establish definitions and boundaries for normal behaviour. But just as the Law adjusts to the nature of crime, just

Illustration for the Book of Job (1825) by William Blake.

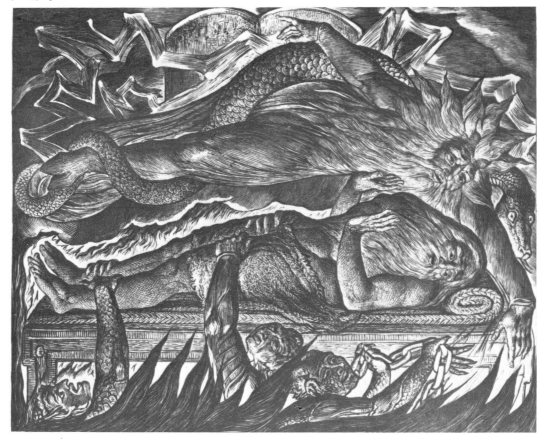

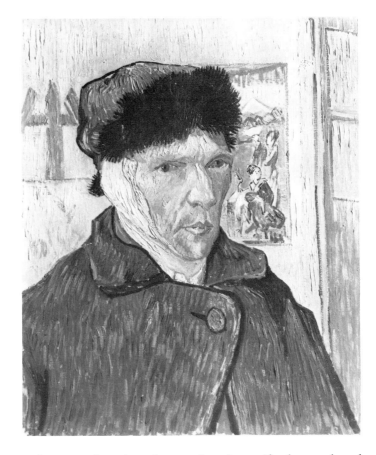

as heretics alter the religion that they offend, so cultural evolution has benefitted from certain extremes of behaviour. Visionaries like Joan of Arc and William Blake, artists like Van Gogh and Edvard Munch, were, by conventional definition, mentally disturbed. The paradox of cultural evolution is that, as it gains from the contribution of those exceptional people who deviate significantly from the norm in intelligence or inventiveness, in artistry or in insight, it also builds up resistance to change, and distrust of extremes, by its emphasis on group identity.

The more revolutionary schools of psychiatry, for example that of R. D. Laing, argue that the definition of sickness of the mind is a product of a fault in society itself. The anthropological extension of this viewpoint

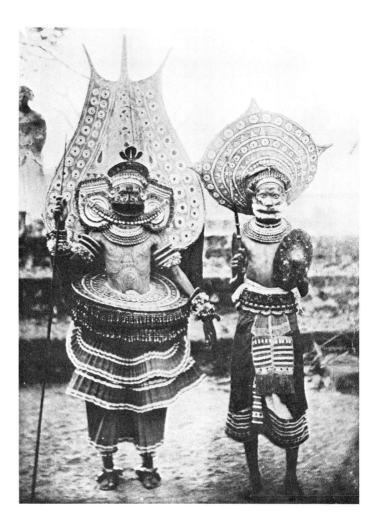

Shaman exorcists in Malaya. Photograph by W. Hutchinson, 1913. There is a prevalent view that shamans and witchdoctors might be people with schizophrenic symptoms who are given useful positions in primitive cultures, where they can exercise their hallucinations and deranged thought processes to the benefit of the community. But this concept, that mental 'illness' is only a label attached to behaviour that is socially unacceptable in developed cultures, has recently been challenged by anthropologist Jane Murphy. She found that Eskimos and Yoruba people do classify some members of their community as mad, but never their shamans and healers. The proportion of the population suffering from socially-debilitating schizophrenia is probably fairly constant in all cultures (there are usually about five to six non-hospitalized sufferers per thousand in the population).

maintains that, since mental illness is culturally relative, those whom we call mad might be able to function usefully in societies that we call primitive. The delusions and hallucinations of the schizophrenic might be admired, and the mentally ill could fill important roles such as shaman or witch-doctor. But recent, careful studies of Alaskan Eskimos and the Yoruba of rural Nigeria have cast doubt on the opinion that the 'illness' of mental disturbance is merely and entirely a label that is tied on socially unacceptable behaviour. Both of these peoples have special names for mental illness, *nuthkavihak* for the Eskimo, *were* for the Yoruba, and

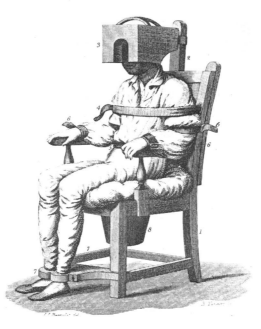

Benjamin Rush (1745–1813) wrote the first American book on psychiatry in 1812. He was generally considered a humanitarian reformer; certainly he tried to free patients from their chains and introduced more active methods of treatment. His 'tranquillizer' was used to restrain the patient while he was copiously bled and purged.

neither ethnic group applies those terms to their shamans and healers. The shaman in a trance is described by an Eskimo as 'out of his mind, but not crazy'. There is little respect for those who are thought to be genuinely mad; they are shackled or sedated by the Yoruba healer, they are tied to posts or locked in barred igloos by the Eskimos.

But if mental illness is not a unique product of *our* way of life, its definition has been stretched to make use of the special powers that society has assumed for dealing with those that it defines as different. In their book, *A Question of Madness*, Zhores and Roy Medvedev give a moving and bitter account of the enforced incarceration of Zhores Medvedev, the eminent Russian biochemist, in a mental hospital, because of his stubborn opposition to local Party bureaucrats and his public pronouncements against the Soviet state. Under the frighteningly broad definition of 'creeping schizophrenia' that is employed by orthodox Russian psychiatry, Medvedev was declared to be suffering from paranoia because he showed 'poor adaptation to the social environment'. Medvedev himself was relatively fortunate; he spent only 19 days in that 'political asylum' before the torrent of protest organized by his brother led to his release. But others are not so lucky; and the abuse of psychiatric definition continues.

Although we are right to be indignant about this flagrant affront to personal liberty in the USSR, we should not believe that our own approach to mental disease is without fault. A lack of sound, theoretical knowledge makes even adequate diagnosis unlikely. In a recent survey, 200 children who had been diagnosed as autistic were subjected to a second opinion. Only 33 were diagnosed as autistic by the second examiner, 53 were said to be childhood schizophrenics, 51 retarded, 7 deaf, and so on.

Just as the criteria for diagnosis are not rigid, so the methods of treatment are largely empirical. The use of surgical damage to the brain in the treatment of the mentally ill is certainly the closest that we come to the horror of socially applied control of the brain, and it illustrates both the inadequate restraints on the treatment of the mentally sick and the poor theoretical basis for that therapy.

In some cases, like the use of the split-brain technique for the treatment of epilepsy, the methods and consequences had been carefully worked out beforehand with experimental animals. But psychosurgery, the treatment of emotional disorders by operations on apparently healthy brain tissue, has proceeded with a lack of experimental background that would be considered inadequate in all other areas of medicine.

The whole of psychosurgery had its origins in a research report delivered by C. Jacobsen and J. F. Fulton at a conference of neurologists in London in 1935. They had been training two chimpanzees to remember where a morsel of food was hidden. One of them, called Becky, was particularly temperamental and became ex-

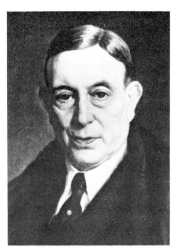

Egas Moniz (1874–1955).

tremely distressed when she failed at this task. She would fly into a tantrum and refuse to perform when the food was hidden from view. Fulton and Jacobsen performed surgical removal of part of the frontal lobes of the cerebral hemispheres (which have rich connections with the emotional centres of the limbic system) and they reported that Becky no longer became disturbed during the experimental task.

A Portuguese neuropsychiatrist, Egas Moniz, rose after the talk and asked: 'If frontal lobe removal prevents the development of experimental neuroses in animals and eliminates frustration behaviour, why would it not be feasible to relieve anxiety states in man by surgical means?' Within the year, Moniz and the surgeon Almeida Lima had started to perform operations on the

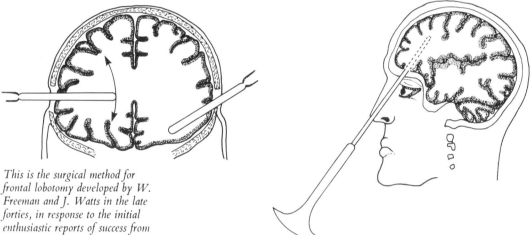

This is the surgical method for frontal lobotomy developed by W. Freeman and J. Watts in the late forties, in response to the initial enthusiastic reports of success from Egas Moniz and Almeida Lima. The diagram shows a cross-section of the frontal part of the head. The surgical instrument, called a 'precision leucotome', was a blunt knife, inserted into small holes made in the temples at the sides of the skull. The blade was then swept up and down to cut the nerve fibres which mainly run between the frontal lobes and the limbic system. This technique was widely used in the early fifties, despite the danger of the 'blind' surgical approach.

Indeed, Freeman, in his eagerness to bring the relief of lobotomy to the largest possible number of sufferers, introduced to the United States an even simpler procedure shown in the second diagram. The patient was merely stunned by an electric shock to the head and a sharp metal 'ice-pick' was thrust up through the thin bone of the roof of the orbit, directly above the eye, by a blow from a mallet. The ice-pick was then twisted from side to side to cut through the frontal lobes. Each side could 'be done in a couple of minutes', and according to Dr Freeman 'an enterprising neurologist' could 'lobotomize ten to fifteen patients in a morning'. Lobotomy was used extensively, even for the treatment of criminals and children, until a storm of protest in the fifties virtually halted the grosser procedures.

179

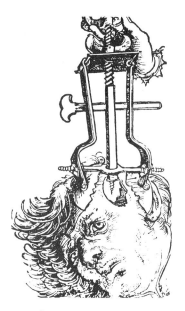

'Trephining' or 'trepanning' was one of a stock of horrifying methods of treatment of neurological and psychiatric illnesses in ancient times. This illustration dates from 1528. The patient was unanaesthetized as a hole was drilled in his skull to release the imagined accumulation of unwanted vapours in the head.

frontal lobes of deranged patients, and by 1950 some 20,000 people around the world, including prisoners and children, had been treated this way. And all of this stemmed from an almost anecdotal observation on a single nervous chimpanzee.

Worst of all, the effectiveness of these operations was evaluated by the very surgeons who had invested their careers in psychosurgery; failure was not easy to accept. And with any treatment for the mentally ill, it is difficult to establish with certainty the success of the technique itself because of the fairly high rate of spontaneous remission from symptoms and the undoubted value of the extra attention that special patients receive, whatever their treatment. However, it became clear that the benefits of gross psychosurgical methods were often minimal and sometimes the consequences were disastrous. Moniz himself, who won the Nobel prize in 1949, was shot in the spine by one of his own lobotomized patients.

But once established, psychosurgery became self-sustaining. It is still widely practised. The techniques are more sophisticated and the surgical lesions much more discrete, but the lack of moral restraint and theoretical background is just as serious.

Significantly, some of the strongest criticism of psychosurgery comes from the behavioural scientists whose experiments are quoted as justification for the surgical methods. Destruction of the amygdala, a part of the limbic system, is used as a treatment for extreme aggression, although in animals damage to the amygdala sometimes *increases* aggressive behaviour, and if it does produce tameness it also destroys the animal's status in the social hierarchy of its colleagues. Aggressive patients have also been subjected to lesions of part of the hypothalamus, dangerously close to regions involved in the regulation of eating and drinking. The rationale behind this procedure is that a similar operation in cats can

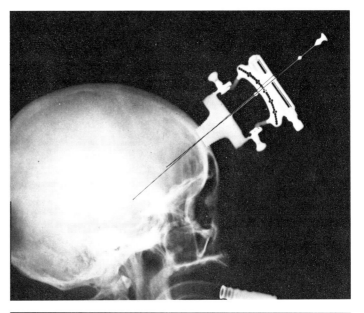

One of the technically more sophisticated of modern psychosurgical procedures is 'bilateral stereotactic subcaudate tractotomy', developed by Geoffrey Knight in London. In contrast to the original, crude methods for destroying fibres in the frontal lobes, Knight's procedure involves the accurate placing of small ceramic 'seeds' containing radioactive yttrium, with a half-life of 62 hours, in the frontal lobes. These X-ray pictures show the aiming device for implanting the yttrium seeds, mounted on the patient's head, and the pattern of sixteen seeds in place in the lower part of the frontal lobes. The array of seeds produces a localized area of radiation damage, about 25 × 15 × 6 mm in size, and there is minimal injury to the rest of the brain. Knight's patients have been assessed by psychiatrists not directly connected with the surgical team (a welcome improvement over previous methods of judging the results of psychosurgery): about half of all patients with severe depression, anxiety or obsessional neuroses showed some improvement, but about one in ten experienced changes in personality or other serious side-effects. Knight's approach is relatively cautious; tractotomy is used only as a final strategy in desperate cases. Nevertheless, it is no more securely based on genuine experimental knowledge than Moniz and Lima's original technique.

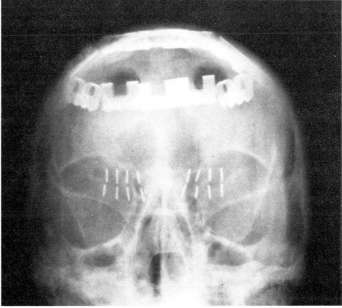

abolish the ferocious behaviour that results from an earlier injury to another limbic structure, the septum. But the septum is not even a clearly defined area in the human brain! Other parts of the hypothalamus are destroyed as treatments for obesity and even a symptom called 'latent homosexuality'.

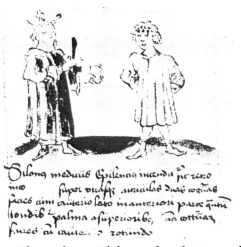

Silong medicus Epilenciu incendu pre vero
mo   super vrurgis aiaurilas due corras
praes aim aurerio lato in anterion parte quini
tondib palma osuperioribc, ma corruas,
fuied ai cauie. o rotundo

Cautery, burning of the scalp and face, was another strategy for the fifteenth-century neurologist. This illustration from Studien zur Geschichte der Medizin *shows cautery of an epileptic.*

That other widely used technique, electro-convulsive therapy, which undoubtedly has brought relief to many of the mentally ill, is nevertheless based on even more obtuse and spurious theoretical justification. The Roman physician Scribonius Largus described the application of an electric fish to a patient's head as a cure for headache, and Pliny the Elder recommended the stunning shock from such a fish as an excellent remedy for the pain of childbirth. But the present-day use of convulsive therapy stems from a revival of the eighteenth-century opinion that maniacs were best treated by a very severe physical stress, and from the entirely erroneous view that epileptics are protected from schizophrenia by their natural convulsions.

Of course, medicine must work empirically until it has sound theoretical grounds for action. Sick people need to be treated. But in most fields of medicine, empirical art has been rationalized, modified or supplemented through experimentally derived knowledge of how the body works. New methods of treatment have grown out of careful and thorough experimental work. In the management of many diseases of the brain this is not yet the case. To that extent, some aspects of neurology and psychiatry are like medieval alchemy practised with twentieth-century tools.

182

It is true that the growing use of drugs in psycho-therapy, which is also not without its critics, has drama-tically reduced the number of long-term admissions to mental institutions. But far more important, the inten-sive research on the action of therapeutic drugs, much of it demanded by law before they can be used, begins to offer hope of an explanation of the biochemical basis at least of schizophrenia.

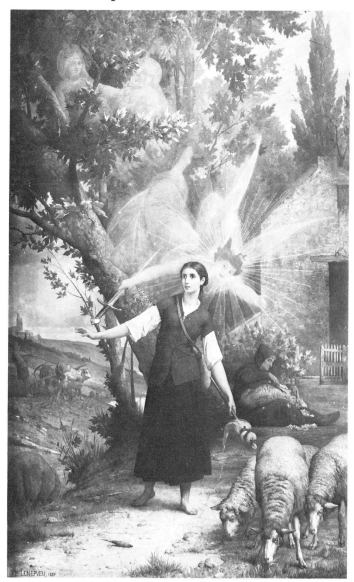

Joan of Arc at Domrémy. Hearing 'voices' is one of the most characteristic symptoms of schizophrenia: indeed clinicians often diagnose schizophrenia on the basis of auditory hallucinations alone, even in the absence of the other common symptoms such as delusions of thought and perception, inappropriate emotional responses and catatonic motor disturbances. Florid schizophrenia is classical madness – the most obvious disturbance of 'mental' function amongst all psychiatric conditions. Yet there is growing evidence that schizophrenia is due to a straightforward physical disturbance of the brain – the over-production of the transmitter substance, dopamine, at certain nerve terminals in the limbic system, the region of the forebrain thought to control emotion. The drugs, such as chlorpromazine and haloperidol, which are extremely effective in controlling schizophrenia, are believed to work by blocking the action of dopamine on nerve cells in the limbic system. The drug amphetamine is known to cause excessive production of dopamine at nerve terminals and many of the symptoms of amphetamine poisoning (as a result of over-consumption of 'pep-pills') are very similar to those of classical schizophrenia.

183

There is, then, the promise that research on the brain will provide a genuine basis for the treatment of mental disease. But much more than that, it will give a greater understanding of the nature of man himself. The study of the brain is one of the last frontiers of human knowledge and of more immediate importance than understanding the infinity of space or the mystery of the atom. For without a description of the brain, without an account of the forces that mould human behaviour, there can never be a truly objective new ethic based on the needs and rights of man. We need that new ethic if we are to overcome the intolerance of difference, which has entrenched society in dogma and discrimination, and to dispel the naturalistic fallacy of arguing that the way we *do* behave is the way we *must* and ought to behave.

I began this book with talk of revolution and I end on the same note. Revolution, social as well as scientific, grows out of knowledge. Only when the choices for action are transparent can proper choice be made. In the words of Mao Tse-tung, 'We can learn what we did not

'The Dance of Life', 1899–1900, by Edvard Munch.

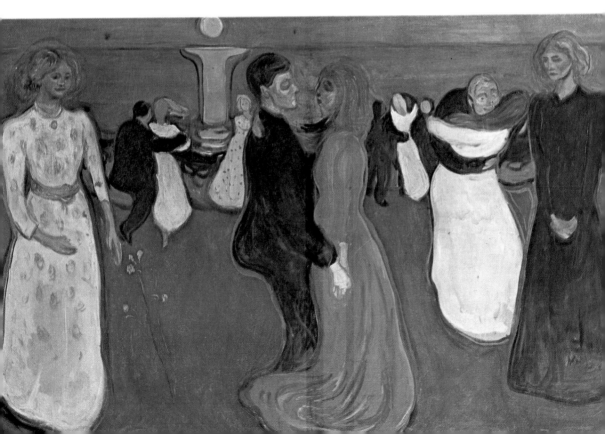

know. We are not only good at destroying the old world, we are also good at building the new.'

I have described the brain as an organ, as a part of the body no more magical than the heart and the liver, which were themselves once thought to do the job of the brain. But also I have tried to show that the actions of the brain are quite unlike those of any other organ, because they determine the behaviour of one man towards his fellows. The brain struggling to understand the brain is society trying to explain itself.

Illustrations: Acknowledgements and Sources

I am grateful to Fiona Hake and Peter Starling of the Physiological Laboratory, Cambridge, for their help in the preparation of several of the original illustrations. Many colleagues, acknowledged below, have supplied photographs and advice about the figures, and I thank them all. But my greatest debt is to Sarah Waters who, with skill and care, researched and collected most of the illustrations.

The diagrams on pages 4, 7, 8 and 17 were supplied by Sandford Publications. These and many other historical illustrations appear in *An Illustrated History of Brain Function* (1972) by E. Clarke and K. Dewhurst. Oxford: Sandford.

Frontispiece   *Water* by Giuseppe Arcimboldo. Kunsthistorisches Museum, Vienna.

Page 2   *Tamping iron of Phineas Gage*. Warren Anatomical Museum, Harvard Medical School.

3   *Phineas Gage's skull and life mask*. Warren Anatomical Museum, Harvard Medical School.

4   *Phrenological map* from *Phrenology* (1825) by J. C. Spurzheim.

5   *Franz Joseph Gall*. By courtesy of the Wellcome Trustees. *Cartoon*. The Mansell Collection.

6   *Lavery Electric Phrenometer*. Radio Times Hulton Picture Library.

7   *Redfield's Physiognomy and Phrenology*. From a description by S. R. Wells in *New Physiognomy* (1894).
Cortical map with phrenological numbers. From 'Della struttura degli emisferi cerebrali' by L. Rolando. *Mem. r. Accad. Sci. Torino* (1830) **35**: 103–46.

8   *Cytoarchitectonic maps*. From *Vergleichende Lokalisationslehre der Grosshirnrinde* (1909) by K. Brodmann.

9   *Anubis* from the Papyrus of Anhai (*c*. 1250 B.C.) The British Museum, Michael Holford Library.

11   *Aristotle* from *Phisica Speculatio* (1557). By courtesy of the Wellcome Trustees.

188

Kunz and H. Fehr. Basel: Birkhäuser Verlag. By courtesy of Dr R. M. Kunz of the Roche Research Foundation.

Page 36 *Freddy, a robot.* By courtesy of the Department of Machine Intelligence, University of Edinburgh.

37, 38, 39 and 41:
Illustrations from *The Expression of the Emotions in Man and Animals* (1872) by Charles Darwin.

38 *Ivan Pavlov* (c. 1904). Novosti Press Agency.

40 *St Sebastian* by Matteo di Giovanni. Reproduced by courtesy of the Trustees, The National Gallery, London.

42 *Acupuncture Meridians.* From the Imperial Edition (1782) of the *Lei Ching.* Kindly supplied by Dr Joseph Needham.

43 *Deaf-mute school in Peking.* Colin Blakemore.

45 *Sleeping and waking brains.* From *Traité de l'Homme* (1664) by René Descartes.

47 *Bes.* Schimmel Collection, New York. Werner Forman Archive, London.

48 *The Ba Spirit over the Mummy.* The British Museum. Michael Holford Library.
Jacob's dream. Bodleian Library, Oxford.
Mohammed's dream. British Museum. Photograph by Ellen S. Smart.

50 *Hans Berger.* J. F. Lehmanns Verlag, Munich.
Luigi Galvani. By courtesy of the Wellcome Trustees.

51 *α rhythm.* From 'The Berger rhythm: potential changes from the occipital lobes in man' by E. D. Adrian and B. H. C. Matthews. *Brain* (1934) **57**: 355–85.

52 *Galvani's experiment.* By courtesy of the Wellcome Trustees.

53 *Hypnagogic visions.* Detail from frontispiece to *Les Rêves et les Moyens de les Diriger* (1867) by Marquis d'Hervey de Saint-Denis. Bibliothèque Nationale, Paris.
EEG records of H. H. Jasper. From *Epilepsy and Cerebral Localisation* (1941) ed. W. Penfield and T. C. Erickson. Springfield: Charles C. Thomas.

54 *Diagram of the reticular formation.* Based on an illustration from *Über der Organ der Seele* (1796) by S. T. Soemmerring.

55 *EEG and eye movements in the cat.* Modified, by permission, from results of M. Jouvet.

56 *Records of paradoxical sleep.* From *Some Must Watch While Some Must Sleep* © 1976 by William C. Dement, M.D. San Francisco: San Francisco Book Company, 1976. Redrawn with permission of the publisher.
Fluorescence micrograph. Courtesy of Barry Everitt.

189

191

cerebellar mossy and climbing fibers', *Arch. Neurol.* (1973) **28**: 118–23.

Silver-stained Purkinje cell. Courtesy of Professor Hendrik Van der Loos.

Page 105 *Electron-micrograph of cat cortex.* Kindly supplied by Dr Laurence Garey.

106 *Descartes' analogy for memory.* From *Traité de l'Homme* (1664).

108 *DNA molecule.* Courtesy of the Wellcome Trustees.

109 *Alexander Luria.* By permission of Professor O. L. Zangwill.
Charles Darwin. By permission of Professor R. D. Keynes.

112 *Peacock.* Photograph by Heather Angel.

113 *Moghul miniature* (*c.* 1600) from the *Akbarnama* of Abul Fazl. Victoria and Albert Museum. Photograph by Eileen Tweedy. Aldus Archives.

114 *The mnemon.* By permission of Professor J. Z. Young.

115 *Jupiter in a zodiac circle.* Villa Albani, Rome. Mansell Collection: Alinari.
Astrolabe by Arssenius. The Mansell Collection.

116 *Alice and the White Queen* by Sir John Tenniel.

117 *Greek and ancient British coins.* From *Organicita e Astrazione* (Milan, 1956) by R. Bianchi Bandinelli.

118–19 *Successive reproductions of pictures.* From *Remembering* (1932) by F. C. Bartlett. Cambridge: Cambridge University Press.

120 *Freeze-fracture electron-micrograph.* Kindly supplied by Professor Konrad Akert.

122 *Flo.* From *In The Shadow of Man* (1971) by Jane van Lawick-Goodall. London: William Collins. Photograph by Hugo van Lawick. Copyright National Geographic Society.

124 *Sulky Chimpanzee.* From *The Expression of the Emotions in Man and Animals* (1872) by Charles Darwin.

125 *Chimpanzees in Norman, Oklahoma.* Institute of Primate Studies, University of Oklahoma.

126 *Neron à l'Hippodrome.* The Mansell Collection.

127 *American Sign Language.* Redrawn from results of Drs Ursula Bellugi and Edward Klima.
Dominus dixit Domino. From the Ormesby Psalter. Bodleian Library, Oxford.

128 *Allogrooming.* From *The Rat: A Study in Behavior* (1975, 2nd edition) by S. A. Barnett, Chicago: University of Chicago Press. Kindly supplied by Dr Barnett.

129 *Narmer Palette.* Cairo Museum. The Werner Forman Archive.
Stele from the tomb of Huntnu. Pushkin Museum, Moscow. The Werner Forman Archive.

193

194

195

Selected Bibliography

References for the sources of illustrations appear under 'Illustrations: acknowledgements and sources'. Many of these also provide valuable background reading.

GENERAL REFERENCES

Adrian, E. D. (1946). *The Physical Background of Perception.* London: Oxford University Press.

Boring, E. G. (1950). *A History of Experimental Psychology.* New York: Appleton-Century-Crofts.

Clarke, E. & O'Malley, C. D. (1968). *The Human Brain and Spinal Cord: A Historical Study Illustrated by Writings from Antiquity to the Twentieth Century.* Berkeley: University of California Press.

Descartes, R. (1664). *L'Homme de René Descartes, et La Formation du Foetus, avec les Remarques de Louis de la Forge.* Paris: Theodore Girard.

Eccles, J. C. (1973). *The Understanding of the Brain.* New York: McGraw-Hill Book Company.

Field, G. C. (1969). *The Philosophy of Plato.* London: Oxford University Press.

Grey Walter, W. (1961). *The Living Brain.* Harmondsworth, Middlesex: Penguin Books.

Hall, T. S. (1972). *Treatise of Man. René Descartes.* French text with translation and commentary. Cambridge, Mass: Harvard University Press.

Haymaker, W. and Schiller, F. (1970). *The Founders of Neurology.* 2nd edn. Springfield, Illinois: C. C. Thomas.

Karczmar, A. G. and Eccles, J. C. (eds.) (1972). *Brain and Human Behavior.* Berlin: Springer Verlag.

Kuhn, T. S. (1970). *The Structure of Scientific Revolutions.* 2nd edn. Chicago: University of Chicago Press.

Lakatos, I. and Musgrave, A. (eds.) (1970). *Criticism and*

the Growth of Knowledge. London: Cambridge University Press.

Luria, A. R. (1973). *The Working Brain*. Harmondsworth, Middlesex: Penguin Books.

Oatley, K. (1972). *Brain Mechanisms and Mind*. London: Thames and Hudson.

Rose, S. (1976). *The Conscious Brain*. Harmondsworth, Middlesex: Penguin Books.

Russell, B. (1961). *History of Western Philosophy*. 2nd edn. London: George Allen and Unwin.

Smythies, J. R. (1970). *Brain Mechanisms and Behaviour*. Oxford: Blackwell Scientific Publications.

Stevens, L. A. (1973). *Explorers of the Brain*. London: Angus and Robertson.

Williams, M. (1970). *Brain Damage and the Mind*. Harmondsworth, Middlesex: Penguin Books.

Wilson, E. O. (1975). *Sociobiology. The New Synthesis*. Cambridge, Mass: Harvard University Press.

Wooldridge, D. E. (1963). *The Machinery of the Brain*. New York: McGraw-Hill Book Company.

Young, J. Z. (1964). *A Model of the Brain*. Oxford: Clarendon Press.

1. THE DIVINEST PART OF US

Bernal, J. D. (1971). *Science in History*. Cambridge, Mass: M.I.T. Press.

Brown, H. M. (1923). 'The anatomical habitat of the soul'. *Ann. Med. History*, **5**: 1–22.

Clarke, E. and Dewhurst, K. (1972). *An Illustrated History of Brain Function*. Oxford: Sandford Publications.

Corner, G. W. (1919). 'Anatomists in search of the soul'. *Ann. Med. History* **2**: 1–7.

Cornford, F. M. (1941). *The Republic of Plato*. London: Oxford University Press.

Harlow, J. M. (1868). 'Recovery from the passage of an iron bar through the head'. *Mass. med. Soc. Publ.* **2**: 327–47.

McCurdy, E. (1907). *Leonardo Da Vinci's Note-Books*. London: Duckworth.

Magoun, H. W. (1958). 'Early development of ideas relating the mind with the brain'. In *The Neurological Basis of Behaviour*, ed. G. E. W. Wolstenholme and C. M. O'Connor. (CIBA Foundation Symposium.) London: Churchill, pp. 4–27.

Meyer, A. (1971). *Historical Aspects of Cerebral Anatomy.* London: Oxford University Press.

Popper, K. (1962). *The Open Society and Its Enemies. Vol. I. The Spell of Plato.* London: Routledge and Kegan Paul.

Sutcliffe, F. E. (1968). *Descartes. Discourse on Method and the Meditations.* Harmondsworth, Middlesex: Penguin Books.

Young, R. M. (1970). *Mind, Brain and Adaptation in the Nineteenth Century.* Oxford: Clarendon Press.

2. CHUANG TZU AND THE BUTTERFLY

Adrian, E. D. and Matthews, B. H. C. (1934). 'The Berger rhythm: potential changes from the occipital lobes in man'. *Brain,* **57**: 355–85.

Coxhead, D. and Hiller, S. (1976). *Dreams: Visions of the Night.* London: Thames and Hudson.

Dement, W. C. (1974). *Some Must Watch While Some Must Sleep.* San Francisco: W. H. Freeman.

Feng, Gia-Fu and English, J. (1974). *Chuang Tsu. Inner Chapters. A New Translation.* New York: Vintage Books.

Jouvet, M. (1967). 'The states of sleep'. *Scientific American,* **216** (2): 62–72.

Kleitman, N. (1939). *Sleep and Wakefulness.* Chicago, Illinois: University of Chicago Press.

Koestler, A. (1967). *The Ghost in the Machine.* London: Pan Books.

Koestler, A. and Smythies, J. R. (1969). *Beyond Reductionism.* (The Alpbach Symposium, 1968.) Boston: Beacon Press.

Lu Gwei-Djen and Needham, J. (1978). *Celestial Lancets: A History of Acupuncture and Moxa.* London: Cambridge University Press.

MacKay, D. (1965). 'From mechanism to mind'. In *Brain and Mind* ed. J. R. Smythies. London: Routledge and Kegan Paul, pp. 163–200.

Melzack, R. (1973). *The Puzzle of Pain.* Harmondsworth, Middlesex: Penguin Books.

Oswald, I. (1974). *Sleep.* 3rd edn. Harmondsworth, Middlesex: Penguin Books.

Pappenheimer, J. R., Koski, G., Fencl, V., Karnovsky, M. L. and Krueger, J. (1975). 'Extraction of sleep-promoting factor S from cerebrospinal fluid and from brains of sleep-deprived animals'. *J. Neurophysiol.* **38**: 1299–1311.

Ryle, G. (1967). *The Concept of Mind.* London: Hutchinson.

3. AN IMAGE OF TRUTH

Adrian, E. D. (1932). *The Mechanism of Nervous Action. Electrical Studies of the Neurone.* London: Oxford University Press, and Philadelphia: University of Philadelphia Press.

Barlow, H. B. (1974). 'Inductive inference, coding, perception and language'. *Perception,* **3**: 123–34.

Battersby, M. (1974). *Trompe l'Oeil. The Eye Deceived.* London: Academy.

Craik, K. (1967). *The Nature of Explanation.* London: Cambridge University Press.

Descartes, R. (1637). *La Dioptrique.* Leiden: J. Maire.

Gombrich, E. H. (1972). *Art and Illusion.* Oxford: Phaidon.

Gregory, R. L. (1970). *The Intelligent Eye.* New York: McGraw-Hill.

Gregory, R. L. and Gombrich, E. H. (1973). *Illusion in Nature and Art.* London: Duckworth.

Lettvin, J. Y., Maturana, H. R., McCulloch, W. S. and Pitts, W. H. (1959). 'What the frog's eye tells the frog's brain'. *Proc. Inst. Radio Engr.* **47**: 1940–51.

Luria, A. R. (1973). *The Man with a Shattered World.* London: Jonathan Cape.

McCulloch, W. S. (1965). *Embodiments of Mind.* Cambridge, Mass: M.I.T. Press.

Moore, G. E. (1922). *Philosophical Studies.* London: Routledge and Kegan Paul.

Penfield, W. and Rasmussen, T. (1957). *The Cerebral Cortex of Man. A Clinical Study of Localization of Function.* New York: Macmillan.

Pirenne, M. H. (1970). *Optics, Painting and Photography.* London: Cambridge University Press.

Pirenne, M. H. (1975). 'Vision and Art.' In *Handbook of Perception, Vol. V. Seeing,* ed. E. C. Carterette and M. P. Friedman. New York: Academic Press, pp. 433–90.

Polanyi, M. (1970). 'What is a painting?' *British Journal of Aesthetics,* **10**: 225–36. (Also published in *The American Scholar,* **39**: 655–69.)

Sartre, J-P. (1956). *The Wall.* Translation in *Existentialism from Dostoevsky to Sartre,* ed. W. Kaufmann. Cleveland, Ohio: Meridian.

Waddington, C. H. (1969). *Behind Appearance.* Cambridge, Mass: M.I.T. Press.

Weiskrantz, L., Warrington, E. K., Sanders, M. D. and Marshall,

J. (1974). 'Visual capacity in the hemianopic field following a restricted occipital ablation'. *Brain*, **97**: 709–28.

4. A CHILD OF THE MOMENT

Bartlett, F. C. (1932). *Remembering*. London: Cambridge University Press.

Borges, J. L. (1967). *A Personal Anthology*. New York: Grove Press.

Hunter, I. M. L. (1964). *Memory*. Harmondsworth, Middlesex: Penguin Books.

Lashley, K. S. (1950). 'In search of the engram'. *Society for Experimental Biology Symposium No. 4: Physiological Mechanisms in Animal Behaviour*, pp. 454–82.

Luria, A. R. (1968). *The Mind of a Mnemonist*. New York: Avon Books.

Miller, R. R. and Springer, A. D. (1973). 'Amnesia, consolidation, and retrieval'. *Psychological Review*, **80**: 69–79.

Milner, B., Corkin, S. and Teuber, H-L. (1968). 'Further analysis of the hippocampal amnesic syndrome: 14-year follow-up study of H.M.' *Neuropsychologia*, **6**: 215–34.

Monod, J. (1971). *Chance and Necessity*. Glasgow: William Collins.

Penfield, W. (1967). *The Excitable Cortex in Conscious Man*. Liverpool: Liverpool University Press.

Pennington, K. S. (1968). 'Advances in holography'. *Scientific American*, **218** (2): 40–8.

Pribram, K. H. (1969). 'The Neurophysiology of remembering'. *Scientific American*, **220** (1): 73–86.

Young, J. Z. (1965). 'The organization of a memory system'. *Proc. Roy. Soc. B*, **163**: 285–320.

Young, J. Z. (1968). 'Memory and the increase of knowledge'. *Nature*, **217**: 905–7.

5. A BURNING FIRE

Brown, R. (1974). *A First Language: The Early Stages*. Cambridge, Mass: Harvard University Press.

Chomsky, N. (1965). *Aspects of the Theory of Syntax*. Cambridge, Mass: M.I.T. Press.

Chomsky, N. (1976). *Reflections on Language*. London: Maurice Temple Smith.

Critchley, M. (1975). *Silent Language*. London: Butterworth.

Englefield, F. R. H. (1977). *Language. Its Origin and Its Relation to*

Thought, ed. G. A. Wells and D. R. Oppenheimer. London: Elek/Pemberton.

Geschwind, N. (1974). 'The anatomical basis of hemispheric differentiation'. In *Hemisphere Function in the Human Brain* ed. S. J. Dimond and J. G. Beaumont. London: Paul Elek, pp. 7–24.

Head, H. (1926). *Aphasia and Kindred Disorders of Speech*. London: Cambridge University Press.

Hewes, G. W. (1973). 'Primate communication and the gestural origin of language'. *Current Anthropology*, **14**, (1–2).

Köhler, W. (1925). *The Mentality of Apes*. New York: Harcourt Brace.

Lenneberg, E. H. (1967). *Biological Foundations of Language*. New York: John Wiley.

Lenneberg, E. H. (1974). 'Language and Brain: Developmental Aspects'. *Neurosciences Research Program Bulletin*, **12** (4).

Linden, E. (1976). *Apes, Men, and Language*. New York: Penguin Books.

Maruszewski, M. (1975). *Language Communication and the Brain*. The Hague: Mouton, and Warsaw: PWN, Polish Scientific Publishers.

Ploog, D. and Melnechuk, T. (1971). 'Are Apes Capable of Language?' *Neurosciences Research Program Bulletin*, **9** (5).

Premack, A. J. and Premack, D. (1972). 'Teaching language to an ape'. *Scientific American*, **227** (4): 92–9.

Skinner, B. F. (1957). *Verbal Behavior*. New York: Appleton-Century-Crofts.

Tylor, E. B. (1865). *Researches into the Early History of Mankind and the Development of Civilization*. London: Murray.

UNESCO (1958). *Japan: Its Land, People and Culture*. Compiled by the Japanese National Commission for UNESCO.

Van Lawick-Goodall, J. (1971). *In The Shadow of Man*. Boston: Houghton Mifflin.

Wazuro, E. G. (1960). *Die Lehre Pawlovs von der höheren Nerventätigkeit*. Berlin: Volk und Wissen Volkseigener Verlag.

Yeni-Komshian, G. H. and Benson, D. A. (1976). 'Anatomical study of cerebral asymmetry in the temporal lobe of humans, chimpanzees, and rhesus monkeys'. *Science*, **192**: 387–9.

6. MADNESS AND MORALITY

Boyers, R. and Orrill, R. (eds.) (1971). *Laing and Anti-Psychiatry*. Harmondsworth, Middlesex: Penguin Books.

Bukovsky, V. and Gluzman, S. (1975). *A Manual of Psychiatry for Political Dissidents*. Amnesty International.

Davies, H. S. (1975). 'Division on the brain'. *The Listener*, 9 October 1975.

Dawkins, R. (1976). *The Selfish Gene*. London: Oxford University Press.

De Lange, S. A. (1973). 'Ethical implications of psychosurgery'. *Psychiat. Neurol. Neurochir. (Amst.)* **76**: 383–9.

Dimond, S. J. and Beaumont, J. G. (eds.) (1974). *Hemisphere Function in the Human Brain*. London: Paul Elek.

Dunbar, J. (1970). *J. M. Barrie. The Man Behind the Image*. London: Collins.

Eccles, J. C. (ed.) (1966). *Brain and Conscious Experience*. Berlin: Springer Verlag.

Fulton, J. F. (1951). *Frontal lobotomy and affective behavior. A neurophysiological analysis*. London: Chapman & Hall.

Gazzaniga, M. S. (1967). 'The split brain in man'. *Scientific American*, **217** (2): 24–9.

Kiloh, L. G., Gye, R. S., Rushworth, R. G., Bell, D. S. and White, R. T. (1974). 'Stereotactic amygdaloidotomy for aggressive behaviour'. *J. Neurol. Neurosurg. and Psychiatry*, **37**: 437–44.

Medvedev, Z. A. and Medvedev, R. A. (1974). *A Question of Madness*. Translated from the Russian by Ellen de Kadt. Harmondsworth, Middlesex: Penguin Books.

Müller, D., Roeder, F. and Orthner, H. (1973). 'Further results of stereotaxis in the human hypothalamus in sexual deviations. First use of this operation in addiction to drugs'. *Neurochirurgia*, **16**: 113–26.

Murphy, J. M. (1976). 'Psychiatric labeling in cross-cultural perspective'. *Science*, **191**: 1019–28.

Ornstein, R. E. (1972). *The Psychology of Consciousness*. San Francisco: W. H. Freeman.

Sano, K., Mayanagi, Y., Sekino, H., Ogashiwa, M. and Ishijima, B. (1970). 'Results of stimulation and destruction of the posterior hypothalamus in man'. *J. Neurosurgery*, **33**: 689–707.

Snyder, S. H. (1975). *Drugs, Madness and the Brain*. London: Hart-Davis, MacGibbon.

Sperry, R. W. (1968). 'Mental unity following surgical disconnection of the cerebral hemispheres'. *The Harvey Lecture Series*, **62**: 293–323. New York: Academic.

Storm Van Leeuwen, W. (1973). 'Intracerebral interventions in patients with behavioural disorders'. *Psychiat. Neurol. Neurochir. (Amst)*, **76**: 345–51.

Tinbergen, N. (1974). 'Ethology and Stress Disorders'. *Science*, **185**: 20–7.

Valenstein, E. S. (1973). *Brain Control*. New York: John Wiley.

Zangwill, O. L. (1976). 'Thought and the brain'. *British Journal of Psychology*, **67**: 301–14.

Index

Figures in bold type refer to illustrations.

208